Using Health Policy in Nursing Practice

Transforming Nursing Practice series

Transforming Nursing Practice is the first series of books designed to help students meet the requirements of the NMC Standards and Essential Skills Clusters for degree programmes. Each book addresses a core topic, and together they cover the generic knowledge required for all fields of practice.

Core knowledge titles:

Series editor: Professor Shirley Bach, Head of the School of Nursing and Midwifery at the University of Brighton

Acute and Critical Care in Adult Nursing	ISBN 978 0 85725 842 7
Becoming a Registered Nurse: Making the Transition to Practice	ISBN 978 0 85725 931 8
Communication and Interpersonal Skills in Nursing (2nd edn)	ISBN 978 0 85725 449 8
Contexts of Contemporary Nursing (2nd edn)	ISBN 978 1 84445 374 0
Dementia Care in Nursing	ISBN 978 0 85725 873 1
Getting into Nursing	ISBN 978 0 85725 895 3
Health Promotion and Public Health for Nursing Students	ISBN 978 0 85725 437 5
Introduction to Medicines Management in Nursing	ISBN 978 1 84445 845 5
Law and Professional Issues in Nursing (2nd edn)	ISBN 978 1 84445 372 6
Leadership, Management and Team Working in Nursing	ISBN 978 0 85725 453 5
Learning Skills for Nursing Students	ISBN 978 1 84445 376 4
Medicines Management in Adult Nursing	ISBN 978 1 84445 842 4
Medicines Management in Children's Nursing	ISBN 978 1 84445 470 9
Medicines Management in Mental Health Nursing	ISBN 978 0 85725 049 0
Mental Health Law in Nursing	ISBN 978 0 85725 863 2
Nursing Adults with Long Term Conditions	ISBN 978 0 85725 441 2
Nursing and Collaborative Practice (2nd edn)	ISBN 978 1 84445 373 3
Nursing and Mental Health Care	ISBN 978 1 84445 467 9
Passing Calculations Tests for Nursing Students (2nd edn)	ISBN 978 1 44625 642 8
Patient and Carer Participation in Nursing	ISBN 978 0 85725 307 1
Patient Assessment and Care Planning in Nursing	ISBN 978 0 85725 858 8
Psychology and Sociology in Nursing	ISBN 978 0 85725 836 6
Safeguarding Adults in Nursing Practice	ISBN 978 1 44625 638 1
Successful Practice Learning for Nursing Students (2nd edn)	ISBN 978 0 85725 315 6
Using Health Policy in Nursing Practice	ISBN 978 1 44625 646 6
What is Nursing? Exploring Theory and Practice (3rd edn)	ISBN 978 0 85725 975 2

Personal and professional learning skills titles:

Series editors: Dr Mooi Standing, Independent Academic Consultant (UK and International) & Accredited NMC Reviewer and Professor Shirley Bach, Head of the School of Nursing and Midwifery at the University of Brighton

Clinical Judgement and Decision Making in Nursing	ISBN 978 1 84445 468 6
Critical Thinking and Writing for Nursing Students	ISBN 978 1 44625 644 2
Evidence-based Practice in Nursing	ISBN 978 1 44627 090 5
Information Skills for Nursing Students	ISBN 978 1 84445 381 8
Reflective Practice in Nursing	ISBN 978 1 44627 085 1
Succeeding in Essays, Exams & OSCEs for Nursing Students	ISBN 978 0 85725 827 4
Succeeding in Research Project Plans and Literature Reviews for Nursing Students	ISBN 978 0 85725 264 7
Successful Professional Portfolios for Nursing Students	ISBN 978 0 85725 457 3
Understanding Research for Nursing Students	ISBN 978 1 84445 368 9

You can find more information on each of these titles and our other learning resources at **www.sagepub.co.uk**. Many of these titles are also available in various e-book formats; please visit our website for more information.

Using Health Policy in Nursing Practice

Georgina Taylor

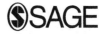

Los Angeles | London | New Delhi
Singapore | Washington DC

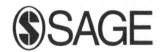 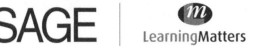

Learning Matters
An imprint of SAGE Publications Ltd
1 Oliver's Yard
55 City Road
London EC1Y 1SP

SAGE Publications Inc.
2455 Teller Road
Thousand Oaks, California 91320

SAGE Publications India Pvt Ltd
B 1/I 1 Mohan Cooperative Industrial Area
Mathura Road
New Delhi 110 044

SAGE Publications Asia-Pacific Pte Ltd
3 Church Street
#10-04 Samsung Hub
Singapore 049483

Editor: Alex Clabburn
Development editor: Caroline Sheldrick
Production controller: Chris Marke
Project management: Diana Chambers
Marketing manager: Tamara Navaratnam
Cover design: Wendy Scott
Typeset by: Kelly Winter
Printed by: MPG Printgroup, UK

Library of Congress Control Number: 2013930253

British Library Cataloguing in Publication data

A catalogue record for this book is available from the British Library

ISBN 978 1 44625 645 9
ISBN 978 1 44625 646 6 (pbk)

MIX
Paper from responsible sources
FSC
www.fsc.org
FSC® C018575

Contents

Foreword

Policy and patient care are directly linked, but it is not always clear to see why or how, and to many nurses health policy is a mysterious phenomenon. Policy directives, whether from local employing institutions or driven by national drivers, can be viewed negatively if they demand changes to practice or additional workload. The benefits may be masked by misunderstanding, poor communication and confusion about the true purpose. This is partly due to the perceived detachment between policy being produced from a wider world view, or by a distant authority and the delivery of care.

Georgina Taylor has written a meaningful text that bridges the gap between policy and the implications for patient care. Examples of health policy are analysed to shed light on the mysteries of policy development, the problems associated with the failure to implement policy, how individuals and groups can become involved in policy development, and then influence the outcomes to positively benefit service users and carers.

In this book you will find understandable explanations of the intentions and potential of health policy. Georgina brings to life the realities of practice and the impact policy can have. You will need to take a leap into the world beyond direct patient care. Once you have made that leap into a world where policy is developed, designed and debated, you will understand the rationale behind important positions taken to protect big issues such as public safety, delivering compassionate care, inequalities in health and improving public health.

As a nurse, if you can understand how policy development and implementation affect your patients, you will be in a stronger position to challenge and develop future healthcare policies that are informed, purposeful and effective.

Shirley Bach
Series Editor

Acknowledgements

The author would like to thank the following people.

- Teaching colleagues in the School of Health and Education at Middlesex University.
- Anonymous reviewers of early drafts.
- Professor Shirley Bach, Series Editor, Transforming Nursing Practice Series.
- Caroline Sheldrick, Development Editor, Transforming Nursing Practice Series.

The author and publishers would like to thank Elsevier Ltd for permission to reproduce (on page 131) the Papadopoulos, Tilki and Taylor model for developing cultural competence, from I. Papadopoulos (ed.) *Transcultural health and social care: development of culturally competent practitioners.* London: Elsevier.

About the author

Georgina Taylor is a Visiting Academic in the School of Health and Education at Middlesex University.

Introduction

Who is this book for?

This book is primarily for students of nursing as they approach completion of their pre-registration programmes. At this point in their careers, nursing students will be thinking about their roles as qualified nurses, which will include translating health and healthcare policy into practice. This book will also be of interest to newly qualified nurses who are experiencing enormous change in healthcare provision as the reforms introduced by the Coalition government are implemented. Registered nurses undertaking relevant continuing professional development programmes or post-registration programmes and those who are 'topping-up' to a degree might also find the book useful.

Why 'Using Health Policy in Nursing Practice'?

There is a tendency for nurses to shy away from policy, but more than ever before, policy that originates at international, national and local levels is shaping the context in which they practise. Many nurses are using policy in their day-to-day practice, but are not always aware of it. Sometimes nurses are knowledgeable about policy, and adapt it to suit their patients and local environment. Sometimes nurses are frustrated by policy. This book takes a practical approach to policy, aiming to raise awareness, to direct nurses to resources that they can use to enhance their knowledge of policy, and to provide examples of how nurses implement policy and how nurses can influence policy.

The book uses examples of reports of failures to care adequately for patients, particularly older patients, though this is done in order to highlight how issues get on to the policy agenda and how such failures then initiate and shape policy developments. It must be stressed that all the reports of poor care acknowledge that good care was also identified. The challenge for nursing is to raise the level of all care to that of the best.

Book structure

The reforms to the National Health Service that were introduced by the Coalition government via the 2012 Health and Social Care Act form the foundation for this book. The content is therefore current, and it is important to be aware that as the reforms are implemented and bed down, the policies may change. Policy is a very dynamic field, and health policy develops at an alarming rate with fast and frequent initiatives. It can be difficult to keep up with it. This book was written after the passage of the 2012 Health and Social Care Act and before the major changes are to be fully implemented in April 2013. It is possible that policy will be adapted during this period. Policy is often viewed as a circular process, like the nursing process, where problem identification leads to policy decisions that are implemented and evaluated. At the evaluation stage, further problems are sometimes identified that then prompt changes. Because of the topical focus of the book, little attention is paid to historical developments in healthcare provision: it is only included when it is believed to be important to set the wider context of the policy concerned. There are plenty of other very good books that cover developments in health policy since the National Health Service was created. It is not possible to cover all policy initiatives and developments, so selected aspects of health policy are used to demonstrate how policy impinges on nursing practice. Two key themes in health and healthcare policy that run through the book are quality and safety.

In Chapter 1, 'What does health policy mean for nursing practice?', we will introduce health and healthcare policy in general, consider the policy process and explore the origins of policy at international, national and local levels. The 2012 Health and Social Care Act is used as a case study to illustrate how various stakeholders, including nurses, have opportunities to influence policy during the journey of policy from White Paper through to legislation. We will also consider some of the critiques of the 2012 Health and Social Care Act.

In Chapter 2, 'Healthcare and social care policy', we explore the increasing attention that is directed to care in the community. Increasing numbers of people living with long-term conditions mean that there are more people requiring support from a range of services that are drawn from a 'mixed economy of care'. We will use a case study of an elderly woman with dementia in order to explore the implementation of policy relating to integrated care.

In Chapter 3, 'The policy context of partnership working', we consider policy relating to partnerships with the voluntary sector, the private sector, patients and their families, and interprofessional working. We will explore partnership working in relation to safeguarding vulnerable people, and in shared decision-making in an end-of-life situation. The chapter is informed by the Coalition government's slogan *No decision about me without me*.

In Chapter 4, 'The policy context of patient and public involvement in healthcare', we explore policy that aims to empower patients and the wider public to have a greater say in how health services are designed and delivered. We will look at examples of degrees of involvement and how organised groups of service users can influence policy. We will also consider how nurses can use patients' stories to inform their practice.

In Chapter 5, 'The policy context of trust and public safety', we will address concerns that led to public safety being high on the policy agenda. We will look at how failure to implement various policies contributed to compromised care being provided to people with learning disabilities in the acute healthcare sector. We will also consider how media reporting of high-profile failures can affect the public's trust in healthcare services, particularly for vulnerable groups.

In Chapter 6, 'The policy context of care, compassion and dignity', we discuss policy relating to caring, considering the social construction of informal carers, and care and compassion in nursing. We explore how compassion reached the policy agenda, and political interventions in what might be deemed nursing policy. We consider the nursing response, including examples of good practice, and the consultation document produced by the Chief Nursing Officer for England and the Director for Nursing at the Department of Health, which presents a vision for high-quality compassionate care and invites nurses to participate in realising this vision.

In Chapter 7, 'Public health policy, inequalities in health and wellbeing and nursing practice', we explore the role of the nurse in relation to public health policy, including policy that aims to help people to live longer, healthier lives. We consider some basic epidemiology, together with the social determinants that contribute to inequalities in health. We explore the role nurses play in implementing policy that aims to reduce inequalities in health and promote wellbeing.

In Chapter 8, 'Using policy in nursing practice', we consider the challenges that nurses face in a complex and uncertain healthcare environment. We explore how policy awareness is necessary in nursing practice and examples of how nurses can use their knowledge of health and healthcare policy. We include examples of how nurses can implement and influence policy. We recognise that not all nurses will want to, or need to, influence policy.

Requirements for the *NMC Standards for Pre-registration Nursing Education* and Essential Skills Clusters

The Nursing and Midwifery Council (NMC) has established standards of competence to be met by applicants to different parts of the register, and these are the standards it considers necessary for safe and effective practice. In addition to the competencies, the NMC has set out specific skills that nursing students must be able to perform at various points of an educational programme. These are known as Essential Skills Clusters (ESCs). This book is structured so that it will help you to understand and meet the competencies and ESCs required for entry to the NMC register. The relevant competencies and ESCs are presented at the start of each chapter so that you can clearly see which ones the chapter addresses. The boxes refer to the latest standards for 2010 onwards, taken from *Standards for pre-registration nursing education* (NMC, 2010).

Learning features

You will find various features interspersed throughout the chapters. These features include scenarios, case studies, concept summaries, research summaries and activities for you to engage in. The scenarios and case studies help you to think about your practice; the concept and research summaries generally help you to understand some of the theoretical underpinnings of health and healthcare policy. Each chapter includes suggestions for further reading and useful websites, so that you can explore the issues raised further. The book cannot cover all aspects of policy, but provides a framework for your learning about policy.

Activities

Throughout the book you will find activities in the text that will help you to make sense of, and learn about, the material being presented by the author. Some activities ask you to reflect on aspects of practice, or your experience of it, or the people or situations you encounter. *Reflection* is an essential skill in nursing, and it helps you to understand the world around you and often to identify how things might be improved. Other activities will help you develop key skills such as your ability to *think critically* about a topic in order to challenge received wisdom, or your ability to *research a topic and find appropriate information and evidence*, and to be able to make decisions using that evidence in situations that are often difficult and time-pressured. Finally, communication and working as part of a team are core to all nursing practice, and some activities will ask you to carry out *group activities* or think about your *communication skills* to help develop these.

All the activities require you to take a break from reading the text, think through the issues presented and carry out some independent study, possibly using the internet. Where appropriate, there are sample answers presented at the end of each chapter, and these will help you to understand more fully your own reflections and independent study. Remember that academic study will always require independent work; attending lectures will never be enough to be successful on your programme, and these activities will help to deepen your knowledge and understanding of the issues under scrutiny and give you practice at working on your own.

You might want to think about completing these activities as part of your personal development plan (PDP) or portfolio. After completing an activity, write it up in your PDP or portfolio in a section devoted to that particular skill, then look back over time to see how far you are developing. You can also do more of the activities for a key skill that you have identified a weakness in, which will help to build your skill and confidence in this area.

Chapter 1
What does health policy mean for nursing practice?

NMC Standards for Pre-registration Nursing Education

This chapter will address the following competencies:

Domain 1: Professional values

1. All nurses must practise with confidence according to *The code: Standards of conduct, performance and ethics for nurses and midwives* (NMC, 2008), and within other recognised ethical and legal frameworks. They must be able to recognise and address ethical challenges relating to people's choices and decision-making about their care, and act within the law to help them and their families and carers find acceptable solutions.

Domain 4: Leadership, management and team working

1. All nurses must act as change agents and provide leadership through quality improvement and service development to enhance people's wellbeing and experiences of healthcare.
2. All nurses must be able to systematically evaluate care and ensure that they and others use the findings to help improve people's experience and care outcomes and to shape future services.
3. All nurses must be able to identify priorities and manage time and resources effectively to ensure the quality of care is maintained or enhanced.

NMC Essential Skills Clusters

This chapter will address the following ESCs:

Cluster: Organisational aspects of care

16. People can trust the newly registered graduate nurse to safely lead, co-ordinate and manage care.

18. People can trust a newly registered graduate nurse to enhance the safety of service users and identify and actively manage risk and uncertainty in relation to people, the environment, self and others.

By entry to the register:

xiii. Works within legal and ethical frameworks to promote safety and positive risk taking.

xiv. Works within policies to protect self and others in all care settings including in the home care setting.

Introduction

Patient safety, quality of care and improving the health of the population are all high on the government's agenda for health policy. In 2012, the Department of Health (DH) in England announced plans to introduce a safety tool to measure basic aspects of patient care – the NHS Safety Thermometer (DH, 2012a). However, these plans have raised questions among nurses and patient groups, because there are financial incentives for acute trusts that choose to use the safety tool (Kendall-Raynor, 2012). The tool requires nurses to record harmful events, such as pressure ulcers and falls, in order to identify areas where improvement is required. Some nurses will question the necessity of these requirements and see this as yet another policy initiative to add to their already heavy workload, but many trusts are already keeping records of this type of information (Kendall-Raynor, 2012). It is an example of policy that has an impact on day-to-day nursing practice. In order to understand policies it is important to be aware of why policies are initiated.

This chapter will introduce you to health policy in general, explaining why policy awareness is important to nursing practice at both micro-level and macro-level. It will outline different levels of policy-making – international, national and local – and relate them to the National Health Service (NHS), outlining the founding principles of the NHS, how these have been maintained over the years and the relevance for current debates. The Coalition government's White Paper *Equity and excellence: liberating the NHS* (DH, 2010a) and subsequent 2012 Health and Social Care Act will be used as a case study to identify the stages at which various stakeholders have the opportunity to comment and thus potentially influence policy development. This will also provide an opportunity to consider key issues that have been raised by stakeholders in relation to the legislation. An overarching policy theme will be that of quality improvement.

Nurses are key professionals in improving the quality of care. The National Nursing Research Unit (NNRU) at the Florence Nightingale School of Nursing & Midwifery at King's College London perceives nurses as:

> *Confident and effective leaders and champions of care quality with a powerful voice at all levels of the healthcare system, from policy-making to the frontline.*
> (Maben and Griffiths, 2008, p6)

Indeed, in recognition of the nursing contribution to improving the quality of healthcare services, the Prime Minister, David Cameron, set up the Nursing and Care Quality Forum in 2012, with the aim of improving the quality of care. The forum consists of nurses from a range of settings as well as patient representatives. You can look at the sort of work that the Nursing Forum is doing in relation to health policy by visiting the DH website (www.dh.gov.uk) and searching for the Nursing and Care Quality Forum. There are numerous other places where you can find information about health policy, for example, the King's Fund, the Royal College of Nursing (RCN), the NNRU and professional nursing journals. You will find some suggested useful websites at the end of the chapter. You can now engage in the following activity to identify a policy initiative.

Activity 1.1   *Evidence-based practice and research*

Search through professional nursing journals, or visit one of the websites listed at the end of the chapter, and look for one example of health policy that might be applicable for your current or recent placement or that is of interest to you.

There is a brief outline answer at the end of the chapter.

Policy in everyday nursing practice

Policy can originate at international, national and/or local levels. Whatever the origin, many policies shape everyday nursing practice. A key overarching and enduring policy theme over recent years, and one that has spanned changes in governments, is that of improving the quality of healthcare. While the emphasis on quality did not originate with the Labour government that came to power in 1997, it became a driving force for the 'new NHS' to be addressed through a comprehensive quality improvement framework (DH, 1997) that remains in place. The concept of clinical governance is central to the quality framework and is defined as:

> *A framework through which NHS organisations are accountable for continuously improving the quality of their services and safeguarding high standards of care by creating an environment in which excellence in clinical care will flourish.*
> (NHSE, 1999, p3)

Clinical governance integrates clinical audit, research, continuing professional development and reflective practice into a systematic framework (Braine, 2006), within which national quality standards are implemented. These standards are set by the **National Institute for Health and Clinical Excellence** (NICE) and are replacing **National Service Frameworks** (NSFs) in the reorganised NHS. NSFs have formed a good example of how nurses can be involved in shaping policy, as they were developed by groups of experts in the relevant field, including health professionals, service users and carers, and other appropriate agencies (Currie, 2000). Clinical governance imposes responsibilities on all healthcare practitioners and organisations to ensure that these standards are met at local level, and also to identify and work to resolve lapses in quality. The delivery of the quality standards is monitored essentially by the **Care Quality Commission** (CQC), so standards are set (by NICE) and monitored (by CQC) centrally and implemented locally by NHS Trusts. Importantly, the ultimate responsibility for the quality of care lies with the Chief Executives of NHS Trusts.

The impetus to improve quality was maintained by the Darzi Report *High quality care for all: NHS next stage review final report* (DH, 2008a), which identified three key domains of quality.

*   Patient safety: first of all, do no harm.
*   Patient experience: including the quality of caring.
*   Effectiveness of care: success rates for treatments and patient-reported outcomes measures (PROMs).
    (DH, 2008a, p47)

The quest for quality improvement has been maintained by the Coalition government, pledging to build on the *ongoing good work in the NHS* through the retention of Lord Darzi's strategy for quality. Spanning the three domains of quality, the **National Health Service Outcomes Framework** provides a set of national outcome goals to direct the NHS. The **National Health Service Commissioning Board** is to be held to account against these goals (DH, 2010a). Echoing clinical governance, the White Paper states:

> *we will create an environment where staff and organisations enjoy greater freedom and clearer incentives to flourish, but also know the consequences of failing the patients they serve and the tax payers who fund them.*
> (DH, 2010a, p9)

Activity 1.2   *Reflection*

Can you identify a quality improvement initiative that is in place in your clinical placement?

Did the policy driver for this initiative originate at international, national or local level?

What factors determine success?

There is a brief outline answer at the end of the chapter.

You might have identified a range of initiatives depending on the nature of your placement, but one aspect of quality improvement, which also concerns safety, is in the area of infection control. This area of practice has attracted policy attention at international levels, for example at the World Health Organization (WHO) and European Union (EU), as well as at national government level and most crucially at local levels where policies are implemented. The NMC (2010) identifies *Infection prevention and control* in its Essential Skills Clusters, requiring nurses to *take effective measures to prevent and control infection in accordance with local and national policy.* So every time nurses wash their hands, use a hand gel or wear a uniform, they are implementing policy.

What is health policy?

Health policy is the term used to describe government decisions and actions aimed at maintaining and improving people's health.
(Blakemore, 2003, p196)

Major changes in health policy might require a programme of legislation at national level, but policy can also result from a statement by the Secretary of State for Health or a speech made by a government minister (Blakemore, 2003). In this chapter we look at policy arising from a programme of legislation that culminated in the 2012 Health and Social Care Act. However, in January 2012 the Prime Minister, David Cameron, made an important statement in relation to nursing policy when he announced that nurses must undertake hourly ward rounds (Triggle, 2012) following a report by the CQC that expressed concern about dignity and respect in hospitals throughout the country. National Health policies .need to be interpreted and implemented locally, but local NHS organisations – for example, NHS Trusts – also formulate their own policies. It is important to point out that, as well as decisions to act on a health issue or problem, policy includes decisions *not* to take action. Health policy also includes decisions and non-decisions by health managers and professionals who make up the wider **policy community** (Green and Thorogood, 1998).

Various models and theories exist concerning the process of policy making, but Buse et al., (2005, pp13–14) propose a simple framework.

*   Problem identification and issue recognition.
*   Policy formulation.
*   Policy implementation.
*   Policy evaluation.

This process is, of course, similar to the nursing process of assessing, planning, implementing and evaluating, which will prompt you to suspect that the policy process is not necessarily linear but cyclical, as policy evaluation might result in further problem identification. In this book you will consider examples of opportunities for nurses to influence policy development at each of the above stages.

A distinction can be made between 'health' policy and 'healthcare' policy. The former relates to policy aimed at improving health, i.e. working 'upstream' (this will be addressed in Chapter 7), while the latter relates to policy that concerns healthcare delivery, i.e. working 'downstream', and essentially concerning the NHS (Hunter, 2003).

The National Health Service

NHS services in England, Northern Ireland, Scotland and Wales are managed separately as a consequence of devolved governance arrangements. The services are similar in many respects, and the core principles of the NHS apply across all four countries of the United Kingdom (UK), but there are some differences and notable divergences (Baggott, 2007). Examples include: the decision in Scotland to make long-term personal care free for elderly people, while it is paid for in the rest of the UK; the decision by the Welsh Assembly to introduce free prescriptions for all in 2007; and the strong emphasis on public health in Wales (Baggott, 2007).

The NHS has been subjected to many reorganisations since its inception, mostly concerning tiers of authority and responsibility. It is important that you have an overview of the structure of healthcare services in your area of work in order to be able to understand policy debates about restructuring.

Activity 1.3   *Leadership and management*

Please use one of the websites below to make sure that you are familiar with the structure of the NHS.

- What are the key institutions?
- What are the lines of accountability?

For information about the NHS in the four countries of the UK, see the following websites.

England: www.nhs.uk
Northern Ireland: www.hscni.net
Scotland: www.show.scot.nhs.uk
Wales: www.wales.nhs.uk

There is a brief outline answer at the end of the chapter.

You will have found that in England the DH is responsible for the NHS, with health services being provided by a series of NHS Trusts, with primary care being the first point of contact to secondary care. The structure of the NHS in England will change from April 2013: the details of the new structure can be found in a series of factsheets on the DH website in the section titled 'Health and Social Care Act Explained' (http://healthandcare.dh.gov.uk/act-factsheets/).

In March 2012 the Coalition government published a revised NHS Constitution (DH, 2012b), originally produced by the previous Labour government. The Constitution sets out the principles and values of the NHS in England and the rights and responsibilities of patients, public and staff. These rights and responsibilities apply to NHS staff and everyone who is entitled to receive NHS services. According to the Constitution, seven key principles or pledges guide the work of the NHS.

1. The NHS provides a comprehensive service, available to all.
2. Access to NHS services is based on clinical need, not an individual's ability to pay.
3. The NHS aspires to the highest standards of excellence and professionalism.
4. NHS services must reflect the needs and preferences of patients, their families and carers.
5. The NHS works across organisational boundaries and in partnership with other organisations in the interests of patients, local communities and the wider population.

6. The NHS is committed to providing best value for taxpayers' money and the most effective, fair and sustainable use of finite resources.
7. The NHS is accountable to the public, communities and patients that it serves.
   (DH, 2012b, pp4–5)

It is important to note that the pledges contained in the Constitution are legally binding.

How is policy made?

Policy can originate at international, national or local level.

International level

There are several international organisations that can initiate health policy; the two most obvious are the WHO and the EU.

World Health Organization (WHO)

The WHO is one leading international organisation that coordinates a global response to the effects of globalisation on health. This globalisation of health problems has come about because of people's increased geographical mobility, international economic interdependence and ease of electronic communication (Bradbury-Jones, 2009).

Activity 1.4   *Evidence-based practice and research*

Please visit the WHO website at www.who.int/about/en and answer the following questions.

What is the WHO?
What is its role in general?
What sort of work does it do?

There is a brief outline answer at the end of the chapter.

You will have found that the WHO has a major role in preventing disease and promoting health, and has formulated strategies for health improvement at a global level and also at the European level through its European Regional Office. We will look at this role in relation to health improvement in Chapter 7. However, the WHO also initiates policy in other areas such as patient safety (WHO, 2009a; WHO, 2009b; WHO, 2011) and a global response to antimicrobial resistance (Campbell, 2007). Moreover, the WHO recognises the key position held by nurses in healthcare settings and urges nurses to engage more in policy formulation and decision-making, while noting that they are often excluded from the process (WHO, 2010). Bryant (2011) acknowledges that this poses a lobbying challenge for the nursing profession – for example, convincing governments of the value of the information and expertise that nurses have relating to healthcare services and patients' needs.

European Union (EU)

The forerunner of the EU, the European Community, was originally established in order to unite the economies of member states, with the ultimate aim of preventing future wars in Europe through ensuring free movement of goods and services and fair competition within a single 'common' European market (Hervey, 2010). A range of institutions make up the EU, and policy making is complex and consists of directives and regulations as well as laws (Baggott, 2007). The EU has limited competence in the field of healthcare as the principle of subsidiarity applies, which means that the running of healthcare systems is left to the individual countries (Duncan, 2002). However, the NHS is affected by EU law concerning the free movement of goods and services, so when a national healthcare system purchases medicines and equipment and employs professionals, the process is governed by EU law (Mossialos et al., 2010).

Since the Maastricht Treaty of 1992, the EU has had competence in the field of public health. This competence was extended by the Amsterdam Treaty of 1997, which required EU member states to ensure a *high level of human health protection . . . in the definition and implementation of all Community policies and activities* (Irwin, 2010, p1). Public health programmes at EU level have included the control and surveillance of communicable diseases, cancer prevention and drug addiction. There have also been EU-level responses to food safety crises, e.g. BSE and international threats to health such as SARS.

However, perhaps the policy that is most familiar to nurses is that relating to the free movement of people and workers, which has contributed to the need to care for patients from increasingly diverse backgrounds and to working in multicultural healthcare teams. EU citizens have the right to work in other member states. The EU Directive 2005/36/EC defines the rules governing the mobility of health professionals based on the mutual recognition of most professional qualifications within the member states (Goddard, 2011). Harmonisation of standards of pre-registration nursing education within the EU has meant that the general nurses' qualification has been recognised in other EU countries since the 1970s (Keighley and Williams, 2011). The Directive was reviewed in 2011, and relevant stakeholders, e.g. health profession regulatory bodies, were consulted on revisions proposed in the Green Paper *Modernising the Professional Qualifications Directive* (2011), and so given the opportunity to shape policy. It is not surprising that patient safety featured prominently in responses from UK regulatory bodies; for example, the NMC's response recognised the valuable contribution of nurses and midwives from other EU countries to the provision of healthcare in the UK, but expressed concerns over language testing and proposed the inclusion of a systematic language check for all EU nurses and midwives who apply to practise in the UK (NMC, 2011). The NMC further proposed that evidence of currency of practice (through validated Continuing Professional Development) is required for automatic recognition of nursing and midwifery qualifications.

National level

The DH is the central government department that formulates national health and healthcare policy for England. The DH provides strategic leadership for public health, adult social care and the NHS in England. It is accountable to the public and to Parliament. The Department is made up of a number of directorates, including the Chief Nursing Officer's Directorate, so nursing has representation at a high level of government.

Policies of national governments are influenced by their value systems. The NHS was established in 1948 under the aegis of the post-war Labour government facing the prospect of rebuilding Britain through a commitment to **democratic socialism**. A key feature of this was the establishment of the welfare state: this government put *the creation of a new and more egalitarian social order at the top of the political agenda* (Jones, 2000, p116). At this point it is helpful to reflect on the founding principles of the NHS.

Activity 1.5   *Critical thinking*

Please visit the NHS website and identify and reflect on the founding principles of the NHS.

Go to www.nhs.uk.

Click on 'History of the NHS' then 'core principles'.

Why do you think these principles were, and continue to be, so important?

There is a brief outline answer at the end of the chapter.

You will have identified the founding principles of the NHS as follows:

- that it meet the needs of everyone;
- that it be free at the point of delivery;
- that it be based on clinical need, not ability to pay.

These principles reflect the era during which they were determined, but have remained very close to the hearts of the UK population, in part due to their egalitarian nature. Whenever a government attempts to introduce major changes to the NHS, these founding principles are often drawn into debates, and we will return to these later in this chapter. But if the values of democratic socialism guided the policies of the post-war Labour government, different values were to guide later governments. For example, the New Right government, led by Mrs Thatcher, which came to power in 1979, espoused a market approach to public policy and a goal of reducing the burden of welfare by *rolling back the boundaries of the public sector* (Jones, 2000, p165). Privatisation and the efficiency and competitive edge of the business world were high on this government's agenda, expressed through the introduction of **general management** in the NHS, the eventual creation of an **internal market** for healthcare through a **purchaser–provider split**, the creation of **National Health Service Trusts** with a degree of freedom from central government control and **fund-holding general practitioners** who were given their own budgets and had the freedom to buy services from hospitals and private suppliers as required for their patients (Jones, 2000). The goals of political ideology often have to be tempered by pragmatism. For example, Mrs Thatcher could not pursue privatisation as far as she might have wished in relation to healthcare, partly as a result of the popularity of the NHS with the British public. Her Chancellor of the Exchequer, Nigel Lawson, once claimed that the NHS is the closest thing the British have to a religion. A change of government in 1997 brought New Labour to power, under the premiership of Tony Blair, with another set of values: the **third way** concerned something in between the democratic socialism of the 1940s and the harsh individualism and market orientation of the New Right. In terms of health policy, New Labour abolished the internal market, the purchaser–provider split and GP fund-holding. However, recognising some of the less divisive benefits of the New Right's health policies, New Labour retained a **commissioner–provider** split driven by *partnership and performance* rather than competition.

The Coalition government came to power in 2010 with the mantra of *Freedom, Fairness, Responsibility* (Cabinet Office, 2010), proclaiming that the days of 'big government' were over, and arguing that centralisation and top-down control had not worked. The aim of the Coalition government is to disperse power more widely in Britain through empowered citizens and communities (Cabinet Office, 2010). The Coalition has meant that both Conservative and Liberal Democrat parties have had to temper their individual party beliefs somewhat in order to attempt to reach common ground. For example, in terms of health policy, *Conservative thinking on markets, choice and competition* has been joined with the *Liberal Democratic belief in advancing democracy at a much more local level* to form a *united vision for the NHS* (Cameron and Clegg, 2010, p9). However, a strong Conservative influence can arguably be detected in health policy, causing some dissent from Liberal Democratic members of the Coalition. While the Coalition government's programme for government expressed the intention to give *every patient the power to choose any healthcare provider that meets NHS standards, within NHS prices* (Cabinet Office, 2010, p26), the White Paper *Equity and excellence: liberating the NHS* (DH, 2010a) elaborates on this theme by promising an information revolution that would provide data on local services in order to facilitate choice and enable the public to exert pressure for unacceptable services to be improved. The assumption is that patients, through exercising choice of where to go for treatment, will drive up standards of quality. Again, this is not a new idea but one that is reminiscent of Mrs Thatcher's internal market.

Theory summary: exit and voice

According to Hirschman (1970), when an organisation's performance is poor, people 'exit' from the organisation, i.e. take their custom elsewhere, or exercise 'voice' and, as customers, express dissatisfaction to those in charge of the organisation. Hirschman (1970, p3) claims that the *decision to exit is often taken in the light of the prospects for the effective use of voice*. In other words, if no one listens to your complaint, you go elsewhere.

Klein (1980) explains how the decision to 'exit' from an organisation does not convey any information to the service provider about the nature of dissatisfaction with the service provided. In contrast, 'voice' has the potential to provide rich information to service providers, and it is easy to see why governments now explicitly adopt policies of user involvement and public participation in order to place service users at the centre of service provision and exert some pressure on service providers to improve the quality of care. However, 'exit' requires competition (Klein, 1980), and the opening up of a market for a range of service providers allows some service users to express preferences for particular providers and to take their custom elsewhere.

Power in policy making

Governments rarely make policies in isolation and have to negotiate with a range of 'stakeholders', raising questions of power: which members of the broader policy community have the most power to influence policy? Several theories abound in relation to answering this question, but two prominent schools of thought are pluralism and elitism.

- *Pluralism* According to the pluralist view, power is dispersed throughout society: no one group holds power over others. The power held by individual citizens and organised groups balances the power of the state, which is seen as a neutral arbiter between different interests (Buse et al., 2005).
- *Elitism* Elitist theories suggest that policy making is dominated by particularly powerful groups. A political elite will hold power and will consist of a network of the most powerful people in several spheres of influence – for example, business and the civil service (Buse et al., 2005).

Activity 1.6   *Critical thinking*

Thinking about the debates that took place as the 2011 Health and Social Care Bill was going through Parliament, which of the above two theories best applies to decision-making in healthcare?

There is a brief outline answer at the end of the chapter.

It is likely that there is a mixture of both theories. In reality, individual citizens and organised groups do have the opportunity to comment on health policy, and the scale of the response to issues raised by the Health and Social Care Bill did force amendments during its passage through the House of Lords. The medical profession has traditionally been viewed as a very powerful group in terms of influencing policy and being quite close to government. The Royal College of General Practitioners had been left out of talks with government since it declared its opposition to the Health and Social Care Bill, but in March 2012 it announced its willingness to work with the government on implementing the proposed changes (*BBC News*, 2012).

Activity 1.7   *Critical thinking*

What other groups of people, or individuals, do you think can be involved in health policy and healthcare policy making?

There is a brief outline answer at the end of the chapter.

Local level

While policy is also formulated locally, this is also the level at which policy is implemented. As one of the professional groups involved in policy implementation, nurses are in a key position to decide how policy is implemented and to report on the process and outcomes of implementation. Nurses, like many other front-line healthcare professionals, sometimes have discretion about how they implement policy in order to meet the specific needs of individual patients and local communities. Indeed, in the White Paper *Equity and excellence: liberating the NHS* (DH, 2010a), it is stated: *We will be clear about what the NHS should achieve; we will not prescribe how it should be achieved.* (DH, 2010a, p7). However, that discretion is always embedded in a structure of rules (Hupe and Hill, 2007) – for example, within professional codes – and nurses can be held accountable for their decisions.

Bergen and While (2005) – see the research summary box – argue that policy guidance is, of necessity, general in nature, providing principles for implementation rather than the detail that would be required for every situation that the policy could be intended for. This can pose problems for implementation. In their exploration of the relationship between policy and practice, Bergen and While investigated the latitude conferred by the vague policy wording and the discretion exercised by practitioners, in this case community nurses who adopted the role of case manager introduced by reforms to the NHS in the 1990s. In implementing this policy, community case managers did indeed interpret policy to meet local needs, moulding policy to coincide with professional nursing values and personal vision. These nurses were operating as 'street level bureaucrats' (Lipsky, 1980).

Research summary: policy implementation in community nursing

Bergen and While (2005) investigated how community nurses implemented government policy in community nursing practice. The changes in community care policy introduced by the White Paper *Caring for people* (DH, 1989) and enshrined in the NHS and Community Care Act of 1990 included the adoption of case management. This entailed placing the management of any individual's health and social care needs with one health and social care worker or team. The research explored how community nurses were involved in case management. A multi-method approach was taken to the research, including telephone and questionnaire surveys and case studies.

The study found that the extent to which nurses adopted and carried out the role of case manager depended on:

- the clarity of policy guidance;
- the extent to which it coincided with professional nursing values;
- local practices and policies; and
- the personal vision of the community nurse.

> **Theory summary: street level bureaucracy**
>
> The term 'street level bureaucracy' was coined by Lipsky (1980) to describe how public service workers translate policy into practice. Following work in the 1970s, Lipsky found that individual workers exercise a wide degree of discretion in how policy is implemented into practice and that they should be viewed as part of the policy-making community.

How can policy be influenced?

While individuals can take up issues they are concerned about with their MPs, probably the most effective way of influencing policy is through group activity. Certainly in terms of nursing, lobbying of governments is essentially the remit of national nursing associations, but not confined to them (Bryant, 2011). In later chapters you will see examples of the work that some organisations have done in identifying problems in healthcare services and getting issues on to the policy agenda, as well as shaping the direction of policy. For example, the Royal College of Nursing was very active in opposing elements of the White Paper (DH, 2010a) and the 2011 Health and Social Care Bill. Activities included giving evidence to Select Committees, holding listening exercises with members and the Secretary of State for Health, publishing letters in national newspapers pointing out concerns on the bill, and holding meetings with senior politicians (RCN, 2010).

In the section that follows you will see how various stakeholders have responded to issues raised by the Coalition government's plans to reform the NHS through the White Paper *Equity and excellence: liberating the NHS* (DH, 2010a) and the subsequent Health and Social Care Bill.

In its programme for government, the Coalition expressed a commitment to an NHS free at the point of use and available to everyone based on need, not the ability to pay (Cabinet Office, 2010). The government also proposed to increase democratic participation in the NHS and to *stop the top-down reorganisations of the NHS that have got in the way of patient care* (Cabinet Office, 2010, p24). There was also a promise to cut the cost of NHS administration and transfer resources to front-line professionals. While there was much criticism of several of the proposed changes, there can be little doubt of the need for the NHS to modernise. The Secretary of State for Health in the New Labour government described the NHS as a *1940s system operating in a 21st century world* (DH, 2000a, p15). However, the Coalition's reforms represent major changes: a journalist (Boseley, 2010) claimed that the Coalition's White Paper would *shake up* the NHS.

When any new government comes to power after a General Election, it will normally have a number of policies it wishes to put into effect. This can often be achieved without recourse to the law, but major changes – for example, the structural and organisational changes to the NHS proposed by the Coalition government – require a change in the law by introducing bills into Parliament. Before a bill is presented to Parliament, there is a consultation stage with those likely to be affected by the bill. Sometimes this consultation process will commence with a Green Paper that stakeholders will comment on. Firm proposals will then be drawn up and presented in the form of a White Paper – the basis of the bill to be introduced into Parliament.

The 2012 Health and Social Care Act

The Coalition government outlined its proposals for the NHS in the White Paper *Equity and excellence: liberating the NHS* (DH, 2010a). This document can be viewed on the Department of Health website (**www.dh.gov.uk**) and the RCN has provided a summary on its website (**www.rcn.org.uk** – RCN, 2011a). In line with its overall policy aim of decentralisation, the government stated its plans to devolve power and responsibility for commissioning services to groups of GPs, i.e. to take over from Primary Care Trusts (PCTs), which are to be abolished by 2013. PCT responsibilities for local health improvement will transfer to local authorities. A reduced role for the DH was announced. Patients are to be placed at the centre of decision-making about care. The key themes of the White Paper are:

• putting patients and the public first;
• improving healthcare outcomes;
• autonomy, accountability and democratic legitimacy;
• cutting bureaucracy and improving efficiency.

In order to illustrate how group activity by nurses might shape policy, the RCN's response to the White Paper is now outlined (RCN, 2010). While welcoming the White Paper's principles underpinning the vision for the NHS, the RCN expressed concern about the lack of detail concerning implementation. The RCN's response to the White Paper concerned two broad areas: supporting the nursing profession and ensuring the best deal for patients. Specifically, this meant: seeking assurance that the founding principles of the NHS would be maintained; seeking assurance that any devolution of powers within the NHS would not result in moves away from national pay arrangements or from national oversight of nursing education and training; urging the government to ensure nursing representation at all levels of the proposed structure; and requesting that the proposed structural reforms would be piloted and evaluated prior to full-scale implementation (RCN, 2010).

Following consultation on the White Paper, the Health and Social Care Bill was drafted and introduced the statutory changes necessary to bring about the desired reforms to the NHS. It is important to remember that government bills are complex documents and that what we read in newspapers and journal articles, or hear on the news, are interpretations of bills. Nevertheless, the critiques are illuminating. An RCN letter in *The Times*, written in conjunction with the British Medical Association (BMA), Royal College of Midwives (RCM) and Unison among others, accused the government of not heeding warnings about key elements of the proposed reforms (Carter et al, 2011).

It is the role of Parliament to see that only bills that are in the public interest become laws. Parliament can pass new laws only when they have completed a number of stages in both the House of Commons and the House of Lords. Without the support of the House of Commons, the House of Lords can only delay bills rather than totally reject them. We will see, however, that both Houses of Parliament can insist on amendments to bills. There is also a final formality when the Queen has to sign to show that a bill has been given the Royal Assent; at this point it becomes an Act of Parliament. The Health and Social Care Bill was approved by the House of Commons and progressed to the House of Lords. Protests against the unpopular Bill by the professional representative organisations, academics, unions and the opposition continued – to the extent that the legislative process was suspended to enable a 'listening exercise' to take place, during which the government consulted widely on aspects of the bill. Several amendments were made, and the legislative process was subsequently resumed.

Several fears were expressed by academics and professionals that the government wished to replace the publicly funded and provided health service with a competitive market of providers, as commissioning groups can contract with *any willing provider* for services (Pollock and Price, 2011; Pollock et al., 2012). Concern was also voiced by the BMA and the Unite trade union over the potential for the expansion of involvement by the private sector in healthcare (Campbell, 2010). Pollock and Price pointed out that the Bill retained the duty of the Secretary of State to promote but not provide a comprehensive health service, raising questions about the future of a comprehensive service, free at the point of need. The issue of the founding principles was also picked up by Ashton (2012), who raised criticisms about the perceived retreat from universal provision, a concept that has been described as a 'social glue' that binds societies together. This is an important function that the NHS is believed to perform. The benefits of a tax-funded health system that provides universal services free at the point of delivery can be illustrated by the early work of Richard Titmuss, a pioneering social researcher who was concerned with social justice.

Research summary: The Gift Relationship

Titmuss (1970) explored the act of blood donation in different countries, and drew comparisons between Britain and the United States of America (USA). When Titmuss's work was carried out, the testing of blood for infections was not as advanced as it is now. In Britain donors gave blood freely as a public service: Titmuss saw this as an act of altruism – individuals giving their blood to an unnamed stranger. In contrast, in the USA there was a market for blood, resulting in paid donors who were sometimes unhealthy people who needed the payment. Titmuss found that, at the time of his study, a private market for blood entailed greater risk of disease to the recipient of the blood than in a voluntary system. Titmuss located the British National Blood Transfusion service within the context of the NHS, which is a universal service and not socially divisive, and therefore fosters a sense of inclusion in society and a desire to look beyond individual needs to consider those of others. Titmuss suggested that the public policy has the potential to encourage or discourage altruism and regard for others through social exchange and reciprocity.

It is this sort of philosophy that people often appeal to when they express fears of the privatisation of the NHS, which could lead to different levels of service for different groups of people, and erode equality of entitlement to healthcare (Pollock et al., 2012).

Klein (1980) described how loyalty to a healthcare system can be generated by equity. Again, this was taken up by Titmuss (1974) in his description of his experience of receiving treatment for cancer at a London hospital. Titmuss describes sitting with five fellow cancer sufferers in the waiting room of the Radiotherapy Department. All of these people had appointments at 10 a.m.

(it was the practice at the time to give several patients the same appointment time). The patients came from different walks of life. Titmuss (1970, p145) describes meeting a young man from Trinidad. He wrote:

> *His appointment was the same time as mine for radium treatment . . . . Sometimes he went into the Theratron Room first; sometimes I did. What determined waiting time was quite simply the vagaries of London traffic – not race, religion, colour or class.*

This experience impressed upon Titmuss the importance of the egalitarian nature of the NHS.

In October 2011, while the Bill was going through the House of Lords, the RCN placed a statement on their website concerning their position on the Health and Social Care Bill:

> *The RCN has serious concerns about the Health and Social Care Bill and the reforms that accompany it. We are one of the leading organisations lobbying the Government to change the legislation to reflect the concerns of our members and their patients.*
> (www.rcn.org.uk)

Politicians also opposed the controversial Bill: Labour's Shadow Health Secretary Andy Burnham pledged to repeal the Bill if Labour were to be re-elected while Leader of the Labour Party Ed Miliband made use of the media to appeal to the public to engage in a campaign to oppose the NHS reforms in an article published in *The Observer* (Miliband, 2012, p8). He argued that the bill threatens the principles of the NHS, and, drawing on the body of opposition from health professionals' representatives, he claimed that *the people who know the NHS best like this bill least.* The controversial 2011 Health and Social Care Bill did eventually receive Royal Assent, and it became the 2012 Health and Social Care Act.

Nurses and health and healthcare policy

In February 2012 the RCN held a ballot of members concerning the government's proposed changes to pension arrangements for nurses, which included raising the age at which nurses would be eligible for NHS pensions. While the majority of those who replied voted to reject the proposals, only 16 per cent of members actually responded, which the RCN found disappointing (RCN, 2012a). It was also a missed opportunity for nurses to exercise their 'powerful voice' on an important policy change that will affect nurses in the future. And of course, governments are unlikely to pay much attention to the preferences of such a small number of respondents.

Nurses have not traditionally been involved in policy making, but it is important that they should be. Nurses need to appreciate the ideas that inform policy so they can understand the context in which they work (Kenny, 2002). Nurses have traditionally focused on the individual nurse–patient relationship and, as a result, have been seen as reluctant to engage meaningfully in the more public arena of healthcare provision (Kenny, 2002). But nurses are well placed because of this established relationship to use the opportunities afforded by an increasingly patient-centred approach to healthcare to develop their knowledge and skills in relation to policy awareness, policy implementation and influencing policy. Indeed, Glasby (2006, p268) reminds us of the increasing requirement for both policy and practice in health and social care to be evidence-based, and presents a strong case for the *practice wisdom of health and social care practitioners*, together with feedback from service users, to inform policy and practice alongside the more scientific forms of evidence.

There can no longer be any doubt that nurses need to be aware of health policy and the way it shapes everyday practice. The NMC has included aspects of health policy in the standards for pre-registration nursing education: educational programme providers must ensure that the following content is included in educational programmes:

*   social, health and behavioural sciences;
*   principles of national and international health policy, including public health;
*   principles of organisational structures, systems and processes;
*   public health and promoting health and wellbeing.

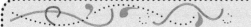

Chapter summary

This chapter has made a strong case for nurses becoming involved in shaping health policy. It has outlined the policy-making process and identified key stakeholders in policy making. The passage of the 2011 Health and Social Care Bill has been used to illustrate how stakeholders can become involved in shaping policy. Several of the issues raised in this chapter relating to how to influence and implement policy will be raised again in the following chapters, which each address a key area within the government's overall policy agenda for improving the quality of healthcare services. The final chapter, Chapter 8, will revisit policy making and engage in further discussion concerning the role of nurses in getting issues on to the policy agenda, formulating policy and implementing it.

Activities: Brief outline answers

Activity 1.1: Evidence-based practice and research (page 7)

There are many possibilities in relation to this activity, but you might have identified a policy initiative that relates to patient safety – for example, infection control – or quality of care – for example, patient dignity and compassion.

Activity 1.2: Reflection (page 8)

There are many possibilities in relation to this activity, but you might have identified an initiative that aims to ensure that the nutritional needs of elderly people are met. The initiative might enforce 'protected mealtimes' when all other non-essential activities are avoided in order to establish an atmosphere conducive to eating and ensure that nurses focus on helping their patients to eat.

This initiative may derive from local policy that has arisen in response to reports from the CQC and The Patients Association about elderly patients' nutritional needs not being met.

Factors for success might include leadership, commitment, organisation and team work.

Activity 1.3: Leadership and management (page 10)

In England the Department of Health is responsible for the delivery of healthcare by the NHS. Healthcare is provided by a series of NHS Trusts.

In Northern Ireland, the Health and Social Care Board answers to the Northern Ireland Executive and works with the Trusts, which deliver services. In Scotland there is a Health Department within the Scottish Executive, which is accountable to the Scottish Parliament. In Wales the Department of Health and Social Services within the Welsh Assembly oversees a series of Boards and NHS Trusts.

Activity 1.4: Evidence-based practice and research (page 11)

The WHO has authority for coordinating health within the United Nations system. It provides leadership on global health matters and has a major role in preventing disease and promoting health. It has formulated strategies for health improvement at a global level and also at the European level through its European Regional Office.

Activity 1.5: Critical thinking (page 13)

The principles are:

- that it meet the needs of everyone;
- that it be free at the point of delivery;
- that it be based on clinical need, not ability to pay.

Activity 1.6: Critical thinking (page 15)

It is likely that a mixture of both theories applies, as several organisations were successful in forcing amendments to the Health and Social Care Bill as it passed through the House of Lords. However, the government remained insistent on some issues.

Activity 1.7: Critical thinking (page 15)

You may have identified a range of individuals, including government ministers, members of parliament (MPs), civil servants, academics and journalists, as well as professional groups such as nurses and doctors. You might also have considered unions, pressure groups, voluntary organisations and patient groups.

Further reading

Ashton, JR (2012) Defending democracy and the National Health Service. *The Lancet*, Early Online Publication, 24 February. doi:10.1016/S0140–6736(12)60287–6.

This article provides a summary of the principles that underpin the NHS and a defence of those principles.

Baggott, R (2007) *Understanding health policy*. Bristol: The Policy Press.

This book provides a detailed account of health policy and the various stakeholders who can be involved in policy making.

Useful websites

www.kcl.ac.uk/schools/nursing/nnru/policy

Policy+ (Policy plus evidence, issues and opinions in healthcare) is a regular publication by the National Nursing Research Unit at the Florence Nightingale School of Nursing & Midwifery at King's College London.

The following websites all provide examples of health and healthcare policy.

www.dh.gov.uk – The Department of Health for England.
www.rcn.org.uk – The Royal College of Nursing.
www.kingsfund.org.uk – The King's Fund.

For information about the NHS in the four countries of the United Kingdom go to the following websites.

www.nhs.uk – England.
www.hscni.net – Northern Ireland.
www.show.scot.nhs.uk – Scotland.
www.wales.nhs.uk – Wales.

Chapter 2
Healthcare and social care policy

Introduction

In this chapter you will be introduced to a case study concerning Ivy, an elderly woman with dementia, that traces her 'journey' from early signs of strange behaviour, through a diagnosis of dementia and her care in the community to her stay in a residential home. You will see how during this journey Ivy was in receipt of services from both health and social services. This is a true story told through the words of Ivy's family, with some narrative from Ivy herself. Ivy's family have given permission to use her story for teaching purposes, and are satisfied that Ivy herself would have given permission; throughout her illness all she ever wanted was to help others. The chapter will use examples relating to integrated care in adult and mental health nursing practice.

This chapter introduces you to the more recent changes in healthcare policy that relate to increasing need for care in the community, the associated need for integrated care and the implications for nursing practice. You will consider the changing demography and patterns of health and illness, noting the increase in the numbers of people living with long-term conditions that can be managed outside hospital but require contributions from a range of services drawn from the 'mixed economy of care' and involving professionals from different sectors. The chapter will use the increasing numbers of people with dementia to illustrate policy relating to integrated care. You will be invited to apply selected aspects of health and social care policy to Ivy's case study, including the *National Service Framework for older people* (DH, 2001a), various documents describing good practice for people with dementia, and policy relating to integrated care. Before reading any further, it is important to be clear what is meant by health services and social care services.

What are health services and social care services?

Make a note of some examples of health services and social care services.

You can draw on your own knowledge and experience, and also visit the DH website. Click on **www.dh.gov.uk** and search for 'Our health, our care, our say'. Select 'Our health, our care, our say – Department of Health Jan 30, 2006 . . . The newly published White Paper'. Click on 'Easy read version of the White Paper', then click on 'Download the easy read version' and select 'Different types of health and social care'.

There is a brief outline answer at the end of the chapter.

Having looked at the range of services that are provided by the two different sectors, you will appreciate that some of your patients require support from both health services and social care services. Glasby and Dickinson (2008) point out that people do not neatly fit into the categories that are created by welfare services, that real-life problems can be complex, and that the people who are in need of a combination of services are often the most vulnerable in society. If health and social care services are not 'joined up', 'seamless' or 'integrated', there is a danger that people will fall into the gaps between the services, with adverse consequences for their health and wellbeing. Successive governments have thus promoted *joined-up solutions to joined-up problems* (Glasby and Dickinson, 2008). While different terms have been used, the DH website refers to 'integrated care', which it defines as *when both health and social care services work together to ensure individuals get the right treatment and care that they need.*

We will now look at Ivy's case study in order to illustrate the need for integrated health and social care services.

Case study: Ivy, Part 1

*Ivy was an 84-year-old widow who had lived alone since the death of her husband, Tom, from cancer. She had been born during the First World War and brought up in the English countryside. During the Second World War she had gone to London to train to be a nurse, and at the end of the 1940s, she had got married, given up work and raised two children, and she had lived on the outskirts of London ever since. Ivy had not coped well with her husband's terminal illness, and, having been married for over 50 years, she was very traumatised by his death. Bereavement counselling was arranged, and a social worker arranged for Ivy to visit a local day centre four days a week. Ivy wore a **community alarm**, which she had first got during her husband's illness. She had lived in the same street since 1948 and had many friends there, though they, too, were in their eighties.*

continued . . .

Ivy had a son who had a young family and lived about 70 miles away and a daughter who lived locally and visited Ivy every evening and looked after her at weekends. The son and daughter decided to aim to do all that they could to keep Ivy in her own home – and in the community she knew so well – for as long as possible.

Over time, however, Ivy's daughter became increasingly concerned about her mother's behaviour. While acknowledging the effects that bereavement could have, she noticed that her mother had lost the ability to handle money and was finding it difficult to make telephone calls. Ivy also did not always dress herself appropriately – for example, in relation to the weather. However, she enjoyed her days at the day centre where the staff were kind and supportive and helped her to adjust her clothing appropriately. Ivy was very sociable and loved company. She attended the art class that was run by an art teacher once a week at the day centre. She loved to draw and to paint; her paintings were always very abstract and always done in bright colours, usually red. When asked about her paintings, she would often reply It's a fierce creature. *Ivy was physically very fit and loved to dance.*

Eventually the daughter made an appointment for Ivy to be seen by her GP, who asked Ivy some questions, conducted a physical examination and did blood tests in order to exclude any physical problem that might be behind the changed behaviour. Nothing abnormal was identified. Ivy's memory continued to deteriorate – she regularly lost her house keys, and sometimes she left the house unlocked, raising concerns about her safety. A neighbour told Ivy's daughter that Ivy had knocked at her door quite late one night and was saying very strange things. The owner of the corner shop told Ivy's daughter that Ivy had been in the shop trying to buy things, but she brought no money with her. Ivy was also becoming increasingly withdrawn. One Sunday, as her daughter was taking her home after a day out and stopped the car outside her house, Ivy burst into tears, crying: I hate this house. It's not the happy home it used to be, full of laughter. *When asked what she would like, Ivy replied that she would like* a little flat.

Ivy's daughter felt that she needed some professional advice concerning the best options for Ivy's future. She contacted the local social services team for older people. The social worker who answered the phone said that social services would not get involved without a referral from the GP. Ivy's daughter again contacted the GP, who arranged for a psychiatrist and a psychologist to visit Ivy and her daughter in Ivy's home – they subsequently diagnosed some form of dementia. *The GP sent a referral form to social services, but no help was immediately forthcoming – Ivy was placed on a waiting list.*

Ivy's daughter arranged for Ivy to spend a trial period in a local residential home. In order to choose a suitable home, Ivy's daughter had sought the advice of the local branch of the Alzheimer's Society. Members of this organisation were very helpful, and while they were not in a position to recommend a particular home, they were able to provide a shortlist of the homes with the facilities that Ivy required. Ivy remained in the residential home, where she was very active, spending her days trying to help the carers, dancing to the music provided by the entertainers, and enjoying days out with her family. She was also allowed to continue to visit the day centre once a week in order to maintain contact with her friends.

The mixed economy of care

Health and social care organisations are under increasing pressure to work in partnership at organisational and interprofessional levels and also with the private and voluntary sectors (Rummery, 2009).

Nowadays people refer to a *mixed economy of care*, according to which services are provided by:

- the statutory (or public) sector;
- the private sector;
- the voluntary sector;
- the informal sector.

The Coalition government's commitment to the provision of services by *any willing provider* gives added emphasis to the existing *mixed economy of care*.

Activity 2.2   ***Critical thinking***

Ivy's case study tells the story of her time spent in the community where she received a range of services.

Read through the case study and identify examples of the services Ivy received under the following headings.

- Statutory.
- Private.
- Voluntary.
- Informal.

There is a brief outline answer at the end of the chapter.

You will have identified that some of the services that Ivy received are provided within the public sector. These are often referred to as statutory services because the state is required by law to provide them – for example, General Practitioner (GP) services, the state pension. Ivy spent some time in a residential home in the private sector. Most residential homes are now run by private organisations following the growth in demand in the 1980s. Voluntary organisations make important contributions to supporting people in the community, and you will have noted the support Ivy's daughter received from the Alzheimer's Society. Community care is also heavily reliant on informal care – the local shopkeeper and Ivy's neighbours, as well as her family.

Origins of integrated care

The second half of the 20th century saw an attempt to develop 'care in the community', which means the provision of health and social services that enable people to remain at home or in a community setting (Glasby, 2007) where in the past they would have been in a hospital, home or other institution. The emphasis on reserving hospital inpatient care for people who are acutely ill can be traced back to the 1950s, when a Royal Commission considered the problems of outdated hospitals providing care for people with mental health problems and the stigma that was attached to inpatient treatment. Hudson and Henwood (2002) argue that the first attempt to coordinate health and social services through national planning systems occurred in the 1960s with plans to replace the country's ageing hospital stock with District General Hospitals; the aim was that people with non-acute health problems would be cared for in the community.

However, attempts to define 'community care' have been fraught with difficulty. A definition from the 1980s conveys the complexity of 'care in the community':

> *To the politician, 'community care' is a useful piece of rhetoric; to the sociologist, it is a stick to beat institutional care with; to the civil servant, it is a cheap alternative to institutional care which can be passed to the local authorities for action – or inaction; to the visionary, it is a dream of the new society in which people really do care; to the social service departments, it is a nightmare of heightened public expectations and inadequate resources to meet them. We are only just beginning to find out what it means to the old, the chronic sick . . .*
> (Jones et al., 1983)

Baggott (2004) claims that the essence of community care is that people should be looked after in their own homes and non-institutional environments rather than in long-stay hospitals and other large institutions. Community care can thus be viewed as a very attractive option if the appropriate support services are in place. However, assumptions have also been made that community care is cheaper than institutional care, and therefore the transition has been seen as a cost-cutting exercise. Implicit in any notions of community care is the belief that there is a 'community' that will care – be it family, friends, neighbours, voluntary organisations – through a network of services including day centres, sheltered housing and meals on wheels. It has never been the intention that all community care needs should be met by the welfare state.

Movement towards more care in the community gained impetus in the 1980s with the publishing of a White Paper, *Caring for people: community care in the next decade and beyond* (DH, 1989). An ideological rejection of institutional care was supplemented by a growing concern about the cost of welfare services to the state. The White Paper formed part of the New Right government's introduction of market principles into the welfare state, and provided the opportunity to reduce entitlements to free care, promote privatisation and shift the responsibility for care to families, friends and voluntary organisations (Baggott, 2004). The White Paper identified local authority social services departments as managers of care for elderly people, disabled people, people with mental health problems and those with learning disabilities (Leathard, 2000). One important provision of the subsequent Act of Parliament (the 1990 NHS and Community Care Act) was that local authorities were no longer required to be providers of care; rather, they were described as *enabling agencies* that were to produce care packages made up of input from a range of public, private and voluntary organisations (Leathard, 2000). One of the key aims of this legislation was to enable people to live in their own homes for as long as possible.

However, as Baggott (2004) describes, there were problems with implementing the provisions for community care. As hospitals discharged people early in order to reduce costs, and long-stay institutions closed, demands on social services departments grew. Although collaboration between health and social services was a key feature of the community care reforms, boundaries that had been in existence between the services since the establishment of the welfare state continued to present problems, and many people who were in need of community care packages fell through the gaps between services. We will now consider an example.

Case study: the Christopher Clunis enquiry

In 1992, Christopher Clunis, a paranoid schizophrenic, without any warning fatally stabbed a young man, Jonathan Zito, who was waiting for an underground train on the Piccadilly Line platform at Finsbury Park station. Christopher Clunis had not been taking his prescribed medication, though he was under the care and supervision of health and social services. A subsequent enquiry into this tragedy identified a catalogue of failure *in these services. During the six years preceding the incident, Christopher Clunis had frequently exhibited violent behaviour, had moved around London, had had several episodes of inpatient care and had lived in various hostels. The enquiry found little continuity of care between individual carers during this time, and poor communication between the agencies that were charged with his care (Coid, 1994). More precisely, Timmins (1994) claims that the blame for the tragedy should be shared by* psychiatrists, social workers, the police, community psychiatric nurses, the Crown Prosecution Service, the probation service, hostel staff and private sector workers. *Further, Coid cites a lack of resources to support Christopher Clunis when his illness was most severe, due to a lack of appropriate inpatient beds. This arose against the policy background of community care, which resulted in a loss of acute admission beds, and closure of long-stay wards in mental health hospitals in Inner London.*

It is important to be aware that murders by people with mental health problems are relatively rare, but this tragedy provides a clear example of what can go wrong when health and social services do not work together. Jonathan Zito's widow, Jayne, provides an excellent example of how individuals can shape policy through her tireless campaign to improve the provision of community care services for people with severe mental illness. She established the Zito Trust as a lobbying organisation aimed at supporting victims: Jayne Zito viewed both her husband and Christopher Clunis as victims of inadequate care (Bowcott, 2009).

Joint working was further promoted by the modernisation agenda that formed part of the Labour government's *NHS Plan* (DH, 2000a), which required health and social services to work together and to pool resources. New **care trusts** were introduced to commission both health and social care in a single organisation. The 2001 Health and Social Care Act gave the government powers to direct local authorities and health authorities to pool their budgets, especially where services are failing.

Why are there policies for integrated working across health and social care?

The continuing political imperative for health and social care services to work more closely together contributed to the overall health improvement agenda contained within Lord Darzi's report *High quality care for all* (DH, 2008a):

> *Partnership working between the NHS, local authorities and social care partners will help to improve people's health and wellbeing, by organising services around patients, and not people around services. This will lead to a patient-centred and seamless approach. This is important not only for people regularly using primary, community and social care services, but will also help people's transition from hospitals back in to their homes. It will also reduce unnecessary re-admissions in to hospitals. In addition local NHS organisations should work in partnership with the local authority, third sector and private sector organisations, patients and carers . . .*
>
> (DH, 2008a, p43)

The background to this renewed emphasis on joint working between health and social care providers relates to changing demography and the increasing numbers of people living with long-term conditions who need care packages with input from both healthcare providers and social care providers. An individual with complex care needs may require support from a range of different professionals employed by different organisations. For example, you will have seen the range of professions that were identified as failing in the case of Christopher Clunis.

The Labour government published the White Paper *Our health, our care, our say: a new direction for community services* (DH, 2006a), which outlined a new direction for community services continuing the drive towards the development of a service *designed around the patient*. This document notes that:

- 90 per cent of people's contacts with the health service take place outside hospitals;
- some 1.7 million people are supported by social care services at any given time.

These statistics remind us that those people receiving care and treatment in hospital represent only the 'tip of the iceberg' of all people who are ill in the community (Unwin et al., 1997). It has been estimated that the number of people over 65 years of age with a long-term condition doubles each decade (DH, 2006a). It is estimated that in England in 2012, 670,000 people have dementia – the equivalent to the combined populations of Bristol and Leicester – and this number is expected to double in the next thirty years (DH, 2012c). One in three people over the age of 65 will develop dementia (DH, 2012c).

The emphasis on collaboration between health and social care agencies survived a change in government. The Coalition government's programme (Cabinet Office, 2010) included a promise to help elderly people live at home for longer with the support of community programmes and a continuing commitment to break down barriers between health and social care. In its White Paper *Equity and excellence: liberating the NHS* (DH, 2010a), the Coalition government retained the commitment to partnership working between health and social services, recognising the interdependence between the NHS and the social care system.

The 2012 Health and Social Care Act contains a number of provisions to enable the NHS, local government and other sectors to work together more effectively. While previous legislation – the 2001 Health and Social Care Act – had made it a statutory duty for health and social care sectors to work in partnership, the 2012 Health and Social Care Act places duties on clinical commissioning groups and the NHS Commissioning Board to secure integrated care where it is beneficial to patients.

Integrated care pilots

Ham and Smith (2010) note the improvements in NHS performance over the last ten years in terms of a reduction in waiting times for treatment and improvements in cardiac and cancer care. They also note that the agenda for the future of healthcare provision includes placing a high priority on prevention of disease, moving care closer to home and addressing the needs of people with long-term conditions. This agenda will mean different ways of working for nurses, particularly because the agenda cannot be addressed by the NHS alone. Ham and Smith (2010) present examples of integrated care pilots that were initiated by the Labour government.

Case study: integrated care pilot

Ham and Smith (2010) describe a pilot of a care trust (a joint health and social care organisation) in Torbay, where integration is based on five health and social care teams organised in localities and aligned with general practices. Each team has a single manager and point of contact. The aim of integrated care is to provide better and more coordinated services for older people who are heavy users of services. For example, intermediate care services enable access to occupational therapists, physiotherapists, social workers and district nurses within three and a half hours if necessary. A unified assessment process and shared health and social care electronic records are in place. This care trust has seen a reduction in the number of delayed transfers of care from the acute hospital to the community, as well as a reduction in the use of hospital beds.

Why should nurses know about health and social care policy?

Activity 2.3   *Critical thinking*

Think about the patients on your current, or most recent, clinical placement. Identify one patient with a long-term condition whose needs are met by professionals from different sectors.

Why does this patient need a range of services?

What is required of healthcare professionals in order to meet this patient's needs?

continued . . .

What is required of social care professionals in order to meet this patient's needs?

Are any other agencies involved?

There is a brief outline answer at the end of the chapter.

You will, no doubt, have identified a patient with a long-term illness, with a mental health problem, or with a learning disability. Your patient may have had a range of services in place prior to admission to hospital, and these services need to be reinstated on discharge. Or your patient may have a new diagnosis and, as a result of this, needs a range of support services.

It should be clear from the above exercise that nurses are in a key position to coordinate care packages that span health and social care sectors. On the DH website it is stated that *integrated care* has the following meanings for frontline staff.

- Working with individual service users to identify the whole range of their needs.
- Knowing what else is available in the system and who else can help.
- Working alongside other professional groups.
- Taking responsibility for bringing in the right care or service, when it is needed.

One key area where nurses are frequently involved in such planning relates to patients who are deemed medically fit to be discharged from hospital, but whose discharge is delayed because they need support in their homes. Since the 1960s, on occasions acute beds have been blocked by the increasing number of elderly patients who, *although deemed medically fit for discharge, continue to occupy a hospital bed because of delays in the organization of continuing care* (Swinkels and Mitchell, 2008, p45), a situation that has thrown into sharp relief the divisions between the centrally funded NHS and locally run social services. While these divisions suit people who need constant medical and nursing care (from health services), and those who need constant social care and attention (from social services), they do pose problems for the growing numbers in the middle who require input from both (Lewis, 2001). Swinkels and Mitchell note a shift in culture away from the very pejorative one of blaming patients for being 'bed blockers' to one that concerns the failings within the health and social care services. While much attention has been paid to the 'provider' views of delayed discharge, Swinkels and Mitchell investigated the adverse effects of delayed discharge on patients, which we will look at now.

Research summary: delayed transfer from hospital to community settings: the older person's perspective

Swinkels and Mitchell (2008) researched the views of older people on their experience of delayed transfer from acute hospital settings in two NHS Trusts in the south of England. Participants were 65 years and over, and a range of reasons for delay were represented, including: waiting for assessment by health or social care professionals; waiting for a care package in their own home; waiting for a placement in a residential or nursing home. The findings revealed that delayed transfer from hospital exacerbated feelings of uncertainty and disruption of usual routines. Participants also expressed concern for deterioration in their condition while in hospital and becoming more dependent; several described themselves as *being busy trapped within my body*. There was a tendency for low mood in older people, and this contributed to them failing to engage in their own discharge planning.

There is a range of government measures in place to deal with 'bed blocking', such as the use of case managers to maintain people with complex needs in the community, the provision of intermediate care services, and legislation that allows social services departments to be charged for hospital beds that are 'blocked' unnecessarily by people waiting for social services provision (Glasby et al., 2008).

The role of the nurse in discharging older people from hospital

When people have to leave hospital too early, they may have to come back again, often more ill than before. The DH (2010b) has recognised that this premature discharge can result in readmission to hospital but claims that delayed discharge increases the risk of loss of independence. As part of its prevention package for older people, the DH issued a resource (DH, 2010b) for practitioners working in acute and community hospitals and intermediate care services to assist the discharge of individuals to their homes and transfer of care between settings. The resource provides a guide consisting of ten steps to achieve safe and timely discharge. Planning for discharge or transfer involves the multi-professional team: *Responsibility for the assessment and planning of discharge and transfer of care must rest with the ward team* (DH, 2010b, p9). However, the role of the nurse is implicated in each step; for example, the first step is starting discharge planning before or on admission, and further steps include involving the patient and carer, and coordinating the discharge or transfer of care process. Moreover, the document states that as the patients' advocates, nurses should be present on ward rounds in order to ensure continuity of information communicated to other team members (DH, 2010b, p10). If a patient is likely to need community care services following discharge from hospital, the NHS has a statutory duty to make a referral to social care services, and this requires the patient's permission. So nurses need to know what social care services might be available and how to make referrals.

While it is essential to be able to engage in safe discharge and transfer of older people from hospital, it must be remembered that there are many older people already being cared for in the community and in receipt of a range of services.

The health and social care divide

Healthcare and social care services have developed from different ideas and assumptions that are reflected in current services (Glasby, 2007). Glasby traces these origins to the time of the Poor Law (in the eighteenth century) when the state first took steps to make some elementary provision for poor and sick people through the establishment of workhouses. Over time these institutions developed to encompass traditional workhouses for the able-bodied poor (who could be 'put to work' in the workhouse) and workhouse infirmaries for the sick and frail. Glasby suggests that this division might mark the origins of the divergence of social and health care, with the poor being viewed as undeserving of support and the sick being viewed as unfortunate and therefore deserving support. The workhouse infirmaries evolved, over time, into hospitals that housed sick people.

The division was affirmed by two important pieces of legislation that contributed to the establishment of the welfare state in the 1940s.

- The 1946 NHS Act, which led to the foundation of the NHS in 1948.
- The 1948 National Assistance Act, which identified the responsibilities of local authorities, including the provision of social services.
(Glasby, 2007)

Under these arrangements the NHS has traditionally provided healthcare services that are free at the point of delivery, and local authorities have traditionally provided social services that are subject to **means testing** (in England). It is this difference that continues to be fundamental to understanding some of the problems attached to integrated care packages. We have already seen how patients who are deemed to no longer require medical treatment or nursing care (which is free at the point of use) can be transferred to social care (which may have to be paid for). If an individual moves into a care home in England and has assets of more than £23,250, they have to pay the full cost unless they have a need for healthcare, in which case the care is paid for by the NHS. Many people have to sell their properties in order to pay for their care. Not only can this be very distressing for patients and their families, who may worry about costs, but some decisions concerning when a patient no longer requires medical treatment or nursing care can seem harsh. The government is considering placing a limit on the amount that individuals will have to pay towards the cost of care.

Once we understand the divisions between health and social care that were created at the time of the establishment of the welfare state, we can understand some of the barriers to successful collaborative working.

Barriers to collaborative working across the health and social care divide

Activity 2.4   *Team working*

Some of the barriers to collaborative working in health and social care fall into the following categories: organisational, financial, legal, professional and cultural (Glasby, 2007).

Considering each category, think of examples of these barriers.

There is a brief outline answer at the end of the chapter.

We have already seen that healthcare is free at the point of use, and social care is means-tested, but Glasby identifies other potential barriers that might result from professional education and training, from policy initiatives that might originate in different government departments and from the boundaries within which the services operate. Whatever might help or hinder the provision of integrated care, such debates are not new. You will see in Ivy's case study that there was no apparent communication between the GP and social services.

Policy relating to people with dementia

We will now look at how the overall policy aims of integrated care are included in specific policies relating to caring for people with dementia. Various policy documents provide guidance on care pathways for people with dementia. For example, the *National Service Framework for older people* (DH, 2001a), *Dementia: supporting people with dementia and their carers in health and social care* (NICE/SCIE, 2006) and *Living well with dementia: a National Dementia Strategy* (DH, 2009a) are important documents. Each of these stresses the importance of a mixed economy of care across health and social services.

The *National Service Framework for older people*

The *National Service Framework for older people* (DH, 2001a) acknowledges that as people age, their needs become more complex, often requiring services from health and social care: *these should be provided in as seamless a way as possible.*

The *National Service Framework for older people* includes a standard for mental health in older people (Standard 7):

> *Standard: Older people who have mental health problems have access to integrated mental health services, provided by the NHS and councils to ensure effective diagnosis, treatment and support, for them and their carers.*

(DH, 2001a, p90)

You will note that in Ivy's case study there was little apparent communication between health and social services.

NICE and SCIE guidelines for dementia

The NICE, in conjunction with the Social Care Institute for Excellence (SCIE), produced clinical guidelines for dementia (NICE/SCIE, 2006 [amended in 2011]). Clinical guidelines represent a major contribution to policy, and health and social care staff are expected to follow these guidelines. We will now consider the clinical guidelines for dementia.

Activity 2.5   *Communication*

Consider the care that Ivy received while she was in the community. Consult the clinical guidelines (NICE/SCIE, 2006), and decide if the clinical guidelines were adhered to. Were there any omissions in Ivy's care in the community?

http://guidance.nice.org.uk/CG42/NICEGuidance/pdf/English

There is a brief outline answer at the end of the chapter.

The National Dementia Strategy

Living well with dementia: a National Dementia Strategy (DH, 2009a) represents the next phase in the government's ambition to improve health for older people, building on earlier initiatives such as the *NSF for older people.* The strategy locates the development of policy and services for people with dementia and their families within the wider policy context, including locating the patient at the centre of care, transforming adult social care, providing a carers' strategy and providing an end-of-life strategy. The strategy stresses that positive input from health and social care services and from the **third sector** and carers of people with dementia can make all the difference between living well with dementia and having a poor quality of life. An ambitious vision of the strategy is a system where all people with dementia have access to the care and support they need.

The strategy stresses the value of early diagnosis and intervention to improve quality of life and to delay or prevent unnecessary admissions into care homes, though it estimates that only a third of people with dementia receive a formal diagnosis or have contact with specialist services at any time during their illness.

Activity 2.6   *Critical thinking*

The National Dementia Strategy states: *People with dementia generally want to stay in their own homes, as do their carers* (DH, 2009a, p34). This statement reflects the continuing aims of community care to maintain people in their own homes for as long as possible.

---

continued . . .

Read through Ivy's case study again. Do you think that Ivy's own home was the best place for her as her illness progressed? What is the role of the nurse in this situation?

There is a brief outline answer at the end of the chapter.

You will have noted that Ivy was finding it increasingly difficult to live alone in her own home. This situation might have been remedied by more support from health and social care services. This is an area where the overall coordinating role of a nurse could be crucial in identifying gaps in a patient's care package. However, you will also have noted Ivy's claim that she *hates this house*, as the home that had once been full of laughter was no longer the happy place it had once been. Her expressed desire for a *little flat* suggests that she wanted to move on, and it might also be indicative of her recognition that she no longer needed a three-bedroom house. Here, again, the role of the nurse is crucial in interpreting policy in relation to each individual patient in their care. People with dementia should have a right to choose where care is provided (Boyle, 2010). However, Boyle also points out that the ability of people with dementia to make decisions is influenced by the degree of support from social care, which in Ivy's case was lacking. While most older people with dementia will wish to stay in their own homes, there will always be exceptions, and the role of the nurse continues to be one of working in the patient's best interests and challenging policy when necessary.

However, government policy in England has supported the development of **telecare** in response to the increasing demand for care services from an ageing population (Milligan et al., 2011), and for those individuals who do wish to remain in their own homes, the National Dementia Strategy promotes the enhancement of housing support, including the use of assistive technology and telecare. While evidence suggests that there are some benefits of the use of telecare, there are concerns among older people and their carers that it should not replace personal contact (Powell et al., 2010; Milligan et al., 2011).

Finally, the National Dementia Strategy provides a care pathway for people with dementia (DH, 2009a, p90). The Department of Health's goal is to help people with dementia and their family carers to *live well with dementia, no matter what the stage of their illness or where they are in the health and social care system.* Key to good quality care is a coordinated and coherent contribution from a range of services. In Ivy's case study you will note that a range of services were involved – for example, the shopkeeper and the neighbours, the GP, mental health services, the social worker and the Alzheimer's Society – but these services were largely working in isolation and not coordinated. Ivy's care appears to be coordinated by her daughter; this role could have been undertaken by a professional nurse from the mental health services.

The way forward for integrated health and social care

Despite years of attention and explicit policy directed at integrated care comprising joined-up and seamless services across health and social care for people with dementia, there is still room for improvement. The National Dementia Strategy was, in part, influenced by a report by the National Audit Office (NAO), which scrutinises public spending on behalf of Parliament. The results of the audits are presented to Parliament, and government departments can be held to account for the way they use public money. The work of the NAO also aims to help public service managers improve performance and service delivery. Following a report by the NAO on services and support for people with dementia, the Chief Executive and others from the DH were questioned on the criticisms and recommendations raised by the report (DH, 2009a). These criticisms and recommendations were addressed in the National Dementia Strategy. The strategy acknowledges that *success will require true joint planning and joint working between health and social care commissioners and providers, the third and independent sectors and people with dementia and their carers* (DH, 2009a, p8). Building on this strategy, the Prime Minister has pledged increased funding for research into dementia as part of his *challenge on dementia* (DH, 2012c), which also focuses on improvements in health and social care, together with the creation of dementia-friendly communities that understand how to help.

There can be no doubt that close and effective collaboration across health and social care and third-sector agencies is necessary in the light of an ageing population and an increasing prevalence of long-term conditions. However, it would appear from ongoing calls for more effective cross-sector working, and increasing academic and political debate, that this is not always easy to achieve.

A report from the Nuffield Trust (Ham and Smith, 2010) suggests that there are several policy barriers to integrated care systems. Ham and Smith (2010) argue that policy makers have given more attention to the development of competition in the NHS than to the promotion of collaboration and integration. Through the examination of case studies, Ham and Smith suggest that tensions exist between the policy of promoting choice and competition, and the policy of developing integrated services: the two policy aims might not be compatible. The competition promoted by commissioning services from *any willing provider* has the potential to increase the range of service providers and thus impede seamless, integrated services. The government has responded to this concern by introducing safeguards to protect patients' interests: **Monitor**, in its role of regulating providers of NHS services, will ensure that patient interests always come first.

Integrated care takes many forms, ranging from care for particular groups of people with the same diseases to coordination of care for individual service users and carers (Ham and Curry, 2011). These authors claim that there is evidence of the benefits of integrated care for older people, and for individual service users and carers. However, they argue that integrated care in the NHS needs to be pursued at all levels to overcome the risks of fragmentation, and of service users 'falling between the cracks' of care. The challenge remains for policy makers as well as frontline professionals to continue to improve the quality of integrated care. The National Dementia Strategy is clear in its aims for effective commissioning for dementia services: at a minimum those involved should include commissioners from health and social services, technical experts, professionals and people with dementia and their families (DH, 2009a, pp80–1).

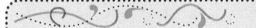

Chapter summary

This chapter has considered policy relating to the provision of integrated care by health and social services working in collaboration. The potential benefits of good integrated care are evident, but the chapter has drawn attention to the lack of effective collaborative working across different sectors. A case study of an elderly woman with dementia has been used to illustrate various aspects of policy relating to health and social care, with particular attention to specific policies relating to caring for people with dementia. You should now be aware of the importance of understanding the various services that might be available to patients who require complex care packages in the community and how these services might be provided by different agencies. You should understand the importance of your key coordinating role in relation to these care packages. A series of activities have directed you to key government documents, and it is hoped that engagement with these activities will have provided some familiarity with the DH website and how to access the complex array of policy documents available. Some of the issues raised in this chapter will be continued in the following chapter, which focuses on policy relating to partnership working. You will meet examples of effective partnership working in order to become familiar with aspects of good practice.

Activities: Brief outline answers

Activity 2.1: Team working (page 26)

You may have found that health services include hospital care and primary healthcare, while social care services include home helps, home carers, respite care and day centres.

Activity 2.2: Critical thinking (page 28)

- Ivy's dependence on her husband Tom is an example of informal care.
- A social worker's involvement in Ivy's care represents statutory care.
- The assessment by the GP and the assistance of the local mental health team represent statutory care.
- The advice from the Alzheimer's Society represents voluntary care.
- In this case, the residential home represents the private sector. The provision of an Attendance Allowance represents the statutory sector.

Activity 2.3: Critical thinking (pages 32–3)

You may have identified a patient with a mental health problem, or with a learning disability, or a physical disability.

You may have identified an elderly person with dementia, a patient who is recovering from a cerebro-vascular accident, a person with a long-term illness such as multiple sclerosis or chronic obstructive pulmonary disease.

You may have identified a refugee, or an asylum seeker, or someone who is homeless.

You may have identified a patient who is being discharged home early following surgery.

Activity 2.4: Team working (page 36)

Glasby (2007, p69) identifies different lines of accountability: health services are accountable to the Secretary of State for Health, while social care services are accountable to local elected councillors; health services tend to focus on the individual patient's medical problems, while social care services tend to focus on the individual in their wider context; health services are strongly influenced by medicine and science, while social care services are strongly influenced by social sciences.

Activity 2.5: Communication (page 37)

You should have identified that Ivy did not have access to integrated mental health services.

Activity 2.6: Critical thinking (pages 37–8)

You should have identified that the policy of keeping older people in their own homes was probably not the best way forward for Ivy.

Further reading

Boyle, G (2010) Social policy for people with dementia in England: promoting human rights? *Health and Social Care in the Community*, 18(5): 511–19.

This article provides a detailed critical evaluation of social policy relating to people with dementia in England.

Glasby, J (2007) *Understanding health and social care.* Bristol: The Policy Press.

This book presents a detailed analysis of policy concerning health and social care.

Glasby, J and Dickinson, H (2008) *Partnership working in health and social care.* Bristol: The Policy Press.

This book focuses on policy and practical issues concerning working in partnership across health and social care.

Department of Health (2012) *Promoting better integration of health and care services: The Health and Social Care Act explained*, Factsheet C3. Available at **http://healthandcare.dh.gov.uk/act-factsheets/**

This factsheet provides details regarding integration within the Health and Social Care Act.

Useful websites

www.dh.gov.uk/dementia

This website includes many policy documents concerning dementia.

www.scotland.gov.uk/Publications/2011/05/31085414/0

This website offers documents concerning policy relating to dementia in Scotland, including the National Strategy.

Chapter 3
The policy context of partnership working

continued . . .

individual situation promoting health and wellbeing, minimising risk of harm and promoting their safety at all times.

By entry to the register:

xii. In partnership with the person, their carers and their families, makes a holistic, person centred and systematic assessment of physical, emotional, psychological, social, cultural and spiritual needs, including risk, and together, develops a comprehensive personalised plan of nursing care.

xv. Works within the context of a multi-professional team and works collaboratively with other agencies when needed to enhance the care of people, communities and populations.

Chapter aims

After reading this chapter, you will be able to:

- recall key policies that promote working in partnership;
- critically discuss working in partnership with other professionals – interprofessional working;
- explore policy and practice in relation to shared decision-making with individual patients;
- explore practice in relation to working in partnership with patients' families.

Introduction

Scenario: Ashur

Ashur is a 33-year-old teacher who has fled the conflict in Syria. He is seeking asylum in the UK – he speaks English fairly well. He has been admitted to a medical ward in an NHS acute trust as his diabetes is out of control. Ashur has told his nurses that he did not have access to healthcare services in Syria; there was a breakdown in local healthcare services as a result of the conflict. He has also admitted that since his arrival in the UK, seeking healthcare has not been a priority for him; he has been more concerned with finding somewhere to live, looking for work and surviving.

The healthcare team have put into place a package of care to bring Ashur's diabetes under control, but are less sure about how to help him with his other concerns. The nurses have advised him to contact the Refugee Council, which has been able to provide advice and tell him about a Syrian Community Group that is forming in his locality. The nurses have also involved the diabetes specialist nurse who, through her contacts with Diabetes UK (www.diabetes.org.uk), has been able to put Ashur in touch with a local diabetes support group.

This is an example of how nurses can involve the voluntary sector in helping their patients.

We have seen in Chapter 2 how many patients need care packages that involve a range of services that may be delivered by different providers, and we looked at the need for closer collaboration between health and social services, and the 'mixed economy of care'. In this chapter we will consider policy that requires nurses to work in partnership with different professional groups within that 'mixed economy of care'; these may be within the NHS or social services. However, nurses are increasingly required to work with providers outside the NHS – for example, in the voluntary and private sectors – and we will look at examples from these sectors in this chapter.

We will then explore interprofessional working, which is driven by government policy on the assumption that it will improve the quality of care. While it is clear that people want to work interprofessionally, there are challenges in trying to cope with a large number of policy initiatives. We will introduce the creation of 'communities of practice' as a possible means of developing effective interprofessional working.

You will consider the tragic case study of Victoria Climbié, who died aged 8 years following ill-treatment and abuse by her guardians. We will look at the failures of communication between the different professionals involved in Victoria's care. This tragic case prompted developments in policy relating to safeguarding children, and you will consider the role of the nurse in relation to this policy. We will also consider interprofessional working in relation to safeguarding vulnerable adults.

In this chapter you will use two case studies to explore policy relating to working in partnership with patients, and the Coalition government's agenda for *no decision about me without me*. First, you will return to the case study of Ivy (from Chapter 2), and follow what happened when she was admitted to hospital in a very frail state and died. You will explore how to work in partnership with Ivy's family in shared ethical decision-making relating to end-of-life care and treatment. Next, we will consider how to work in partnership with Sharon, a woman with multiple sclerosis, in order to maintain her usual routines when she is admitted to hospital with a chest infection.

Partnership working: the policy context

Issues relating to developing interprofessional partnerships and promoting partnerships between different agencies can be found in policy documents since the 1960s, but partnership working was given greater impetus during the 1980s. Drivers of government policy on interprofessional working include the complexity and increasing cost of caring for people with long-term conditions. Closer collaboration between different professionals was implicit in the provisions of the 1990 NHS and Community Care Act, which required local authorities to publish community care plans and to consult with users of services and a range of local agencies, including health authorities, housing departments, the voluntary and private sector and informal carers (Leathard, 2003, p20). In 1997 the New Labour government gave primacy to joint working in public services, and conveyed this via the White Paper *The new NHS: modern, dependable* (DH, 1997). Collaboration was central to the modernisation agenda, which embraced a *third way* of running the NHS, based on *partnership and performance* rather than the competitive approach adopted by the previous New Right governments. Partnership was to be achieved by placing the patient at the centre of the care process. Hudson (1998, pp30–1) identified five partnership approaches in the White Paper.

- Programme partnership: programmes that aimed to tackle the causes of ill health featured prominently. Examples included **Health Improvement Programmes** (HImPs) and **Health Action Zones** (HAZs). Both programmes aimed to improve the health of local populations through partnerships between hospitals, GPs, local authorities, voluntary organisations and local businesses.
- Professional partnerships: NHS staff were required to work as interprofessional teams within the health sector and to work across organisational boundaries.
- Administrative partnerships: Primary Care Groups were expected to work closely with social services in planning and delivering services.
- Performance partnership: A new national performance framework required regional NHS and social services offices to work closely together.
- Governance partnership: in order to address the **'democratic deficit'** representatives from local communities were to be included on NHS Boards.

Other policy documents that employed the vocabulary of collaboration included *A first class service: quality in the new NHS* (DH, 1998a) and *Clinical governance: quality in the new NHS* (NHSE, 1999), which both required professionals to work together across traditional boundaries (Kenny, 2002). The Labour government explicitly maintained this approach in its White Paper *Our health, our care, our say* (DH, 2006a), and launched the Social Enterprise Unit in the DH in 2006, which invited health and/or social care staff and multi-agency partnerships to set up innovative **social enterprises** that would be tailored to the needs of their local communities. Social enterprises are becoming increasingly common as providers of NHS services within the mixed economy of care (Cheater, 2010); the following case study describes one example.

Case study: social enterprise

The East London Wound Healing Centre comprises a wound care and lymphoedema nurse-led team as well as a multidisciplinary team. The centre re-launched as the Accelerate Community Interest Company, a social enterprise, continuing its previous role of offering advice to community nursing teams, primary care and nursing homes. Early indications are that the team now feels free to be more creative and is able to provide care that is more tailored to the needs of its clients (Hopkins, 2012).

This is an example of nurses responding to government policy relating to innovative ways of working within the mixed economy of care and how nurses can set up a business to work in partnership with the NHS. However, Gillen (2010) warns prospective nurse entrepreneurs that social enterprise staff are not employed by the NHS and therefore not entitled to the benefits of NHS employment, and Cheater (2010) reports that there is little evidence of the impact of nurse-led social enterprises on improving care. Working in partnership with the voluntary and private sectors and encouraging social enterprises are included in the policies of the Coalition government – the provision of healthcare and social services is no longer confined to the public sector.

Partnership working with the voluntary sector

The voluntary sector was active in providing health and social services before the creation of the NHS, which took over most of their functions in order to provide a universal and comprehensive service. Nevertheless, the voluntary sector has continued to provide valuable services, particularly for vulnerable groups of people.

Activity 3.1   *Team working*

Which voluntary organisations are you familiar with?

Choose one of these organisations and make brief notes about the role it performs.

Can you think of any voluntary organisations that nurses might engage with?

There is a brief outline answer at the end of the chapter.

The possibilities for contact with voluntary sector organisations are numerous. One example you might have chosen is the British Red Cross (www.redcross.org.uk). As well as their well-publicised responses to world disasters, Red Cross volunteers provide vital work to support healthcare provision in the community. For example, there is a scheme that provides volunteers to visit people in their homes following a short stay in hospital and help them to readjust to life at home. These volunteers do not perform nursing duties, but provide practical help such as shopping, as well as companionship. The Red Cross also provides short-term loans of medical equipment such as wheelchairs. Referrals for these services come from GPs, hospitals and social workers as well as individuals.

Alternatively, you might have chosen one of the many voluntary organisations that provide information for people with particular disorders, for example, the British Heart Foundation (www.bhf.org.uk). Or, you might have chosen a voluntary organisation that helps particular groups of people, for example the Refugee Council (www.refugeecouncil.org.uk), which provides information, advice and support to refugees and asylum seekers, as seen in the scenario provided at the beginning of this chapter.

Partnership working with the private sector

There has always been some private provision of healthcare alongside the public sector provision by the NHS. Since the 1980s and 1990s, the NHS has been encouraged to use the private sector for selected treatments (funded by the NHS) in order to reduce waiting lists (Glasby, 2007). Some private sector companies won contracts to deliver ancillary services, such as cleaning and catering. Some controversies have arisen because the private sector often aims to make a profit, an approach that can hinder partnership working with the public sector, which does not normally make a profit.

In the 1990s **Private Finance Initiatives** (PFIs) were introduced, which allow private companies to design, finance and build new hospitals (Glasby, 2007). The private companies charge the NHS an annual fee, usually over a thirty-year term. PFIs have become very controversial as they are proving to be very costly to NHS trusts. The *Nursing Standard* reports that a *burden of debt* is bringing NHS trusts close to collapse (*Nursing Standard*, 2011, p10). New Labour, under the premiership of Tony Blair, continued with PFIs under its public–private partnership programme, and further encouraged use of the private sector to reduce waiting times and waiting lists for treatments. New Labour also initiated **Independent Sector Treatment Centres** (ISTCs) to undertake work on behalf of the NHS (Glasby, 2007). These developments have given the private sector a significant role in the provision of healthcare, and this trend continues under the Coalition government.

Working in partnership with the private sector can produce positive results. Pallister and Lavin (2010) report on partnership working between primary care and a commercial organisation, Slimming World, that helps obese and overweight patients to lose weight and improve their lifestyle. The service is coordinated by practice nurses who identify patients who might be suitable for the service, discuss weight management with them, refer them to the service and monitor their progress. PCTs fund places on the programme; patients are given vouchers to join a Slimming World group of their choice, where they are given advice about a healthy balanced diet and suitable activity that is in line with government recommendations. The programme conforms to NICE guidelines (CG43) for obesity (NICE, 2006a), and the outcomes are encouraging.

Partnership working with other professionals

Interprofessional working requires that personnel from different professions and agencies work together.
(Pollard et al., 2005, p6)

As Meads and Ashcroft (2005) point out, care management, individual needs assessments and care pathways all require interprofessional collaboration if they are to be successful. This view is reflected in government policies that demand seamless, 'joined-up' health and social care services that are more responsive to each other and to service users. As such, the government is the central driver for interprofessional working, which occurs within health services as well as with other agencies. You can now consider working with other professionals within the NHS.

Activity 3.2   *Team working*

Think about your current or recent clinical placement.

Which other professionals did you work with?

What circumstances required you to work collaboratively with these professionals?

There is a brief outline answer at the end of the chapter.

Effective interprofessional working requires a commitment to equality and collective responsibility and the removal of traditional hierarchies. Scott et al. (2005) identify how communication problems can arise between members of the same profession, e.g. consultants and junior doctors, hospital and community nurses, as well as with other professions. However, Kenny (2002) highlights some contradictions in policy. While interprofessional working is central to clinical governance, policy has suggested that the lead for clinical governance should be taken by a medical director (Kenny, 2002). If joint working is to become a reality, the dominance by medical practitioners must change (Baxter and Brumfitt, 2008).

Research summary: professional differences in interprofessional working

Baxter and Brumfitt (2008) report on a case study that examined joint working among staff providing services to stroke patients. The aim was to explore factors that affected joint working. The research revealed three factors that are significant in interprofessional working.

- Professional knowledge and skills.
- Professional role and identity.
- Power and status.

The findings revealed that role boundaries were maintained through profession-specific knowledge and skills, though some exchange of knowledge and skills was evident; for example, a speech and language therapist said: *the people here were available to have their brains picked and then we started to problem solve together* (Baxter and Brumfitt, 2008, p243). There was some variation among staff concerning whether they saw their identity as a member of their profession or as a member of the multidisciplinary team. Professional identities were strong, with awareness of professional roles and duties of care. While there were perceptions of the power of medical staff in decision-making, in reality other health professionals were able to influence decision-making.

This research demonstrates that, despite the promotion of interprofessional working by government policies, strong professional identities have the potential to impede joint working. At the same time, however, for interprofessional working to be successful, it is important that individual professionals are very secure in their own particular role within the team. The above study concerned the care of patients who had suffered strokes; the progression of care pathways following a stroke entails working with the patient towards increasing independence, so there is heavy reliance on a range of different professionals – such as occupational therapists, speech therapists and physiotherapists, as well as nurses – working closely together and sharing their expertise. In this case the professionals were all working within the health service; interprofessional working can become more complex when professionals have to work with services outside the health service.

There is an assumption that interprofessional working will improve the quality of services delivered (Barrett et al., 2005). Against the background of critiques of this policy assumption, Hingley-Jones and Allain (2008) explore the process of service integration for disabled children and their families.

Research summary: integrating services for disabled children and their families in two English local authorities

Hingley-Jones and Allain (2008) used semi-structured interviews with professionals from health, social care and education, as well as with representatives from parent-carer groups and voluntary agencies, to explore the structuring of services for disabled children and their families, and understanding and interpretation of policy developments concerning integration of services.

The researchers found evidence of efforts being made to consult with disabled children and their families on the shaping of services. However, some parents and carers experienced difficulties in dealing with multi-professional groups. Professionals were moving towards integrated services, though they were troubled by other policy developments – for example, budgetary cuts, which made staff fear losing their jobs. Professional informants were optimistic about developing interprofessional services within recently established Children's Trusts, though there were elements of professional rivalry, and professional differences in relation to values and language.

Safeguarding children

While individual professionals are accountable for their own actions, interprofessional working implies accountability for the overall programmes they participate in (Meads and Ashcroft, 2005). Failures in interprofessional working can result in very serious consequences, as identified in the Kennedy Report (Kennedy, 2001) into the high mortality rate of children undergoing paediatric cardiac surgery at the United Bristol Hospital Trust, and the Laming Report (DH, 2003) into the death of Victoria Climbié. Both reports identified poor communication, poor interprofessional working and poor teamwork, among other contributory factors. We have seen in Chapter 2 how health and social care services need to work more closely together to provide holistic packages of care. Now we will consider the case study of Victoria Climbié, looking at how different professions failed to communicate efficiently across health, social and police services, and how such failings contributed to the tragic death of Victoria, and subsequently to a public inquiry. The findings of the public inquiry then prompted a series of policy developments on safeguarding children.

Case study: Victoria Climbié

Victoria Climbié was a young African girl who came to England from the Ivory Coast with her great-aunt in 1999. Victoria's parents believed that she would have a better education and life in Europe. Victoria suffered months of severe ill-treatment and abuse from her great-aunt and her partner, resulting in Victoria's death in 2000 from multiple injuries – she was 8 years old. Victoria's great-aunt and her partner were convicted of Victoria's murder. Soon after arrival in England, while they were in temporary housing, concerns were raised by a relative of her great-aunt about Victoria's welfare. Social services were alerted, and signs of a child in need were detected. However, the subsequent referral was badly handled, and the case was not followed up satisfactorily.

Victoria's childminder's daughter took Victoria to hospital because of injuries on her body, and Victoria was admitted to hospital because of the strong possibility of non-accidental injury. As it was believed that she had suffered abuse, a referral was made to social services, and she was placed under police protection. Subsequently another doctor diagnosed scabies, and the police protection was withdrawn. The great-aunt discharged Victoria from hospital the following day, and the abuse issues were not followed up. A week later Victoria was admitted to another hospital with a scald on her face, and clinicians had concerns about her. She was referred to social services, and a social worker was allocated to her; she was discharged back to the care of her great-aunt. The inquiry found poor communication between hospital and social services with a lack of recorded information. Victoria later died from continuing abuse.
(DH, 2003)

There was a network of organisations and individual professionals who had contact with Victoria, including a local authority housing department, social services, the police and two hospitals. The public inquiry found that there were at least twelve occasions when opportunities arose to help Victoria and that the failures to use the opportunities were the result of ineffective inter-professional and inter-agency working. As well as failure of communication between different staff and agencies, the public inquiry identified that *widespread organisational malaise* contributed to the poor information exchange. Further, there was a failure to follow established procedures. In spite of the existence of policy promoting collaborative working to promote children's welfare and protect them from abuse, there was poor implementation of the provisions of the Children Act 1989.

The public inquiry into this tragedy influenced policy relating to children's services – for example, the establishment of new service arrangements such as local Children's Trusts where multi-disciplinary teams from health, education and social services are brought together (Scott et al., 2005). Further policy developments included the Green Paper *Every child matters* (Department for

Education and Skills, 2003), the Children Act 2004 and Local Safeguarding Children's Boards. The government also produced guidance on inter-agency working to protect children, including a common assessment framework (CAF), which provides a structure for a written referral. It also stresses the importance of documentation when making referrals, when having discussions with other professionals and when decisions are made.

Nevertheless, while policy to protect children is in place, abuse of children continues. In 2008 Peter Connelly (originally referred to as Baby P) a 17-month-old toddler died following non-accidental injuries. Lord Laming was asked to conduct a review of child protection procedures, and consequently government child protection guidance – *Working together to safeguard children* (Department for Education, 2010) – was strengthened. Lord Laming concluded that policy exists to safeguard children but that there are failures to implement policy – for example, concerning the use of the CAF.

Safeguarding and promoting the welfare of children is the responsibility of the local authority, working in partnership with other public organisations, healthcare professionals, the voluntary sector, children and young people, parents, carers and the wider community. Nurses – wherever they work and in their private lives – have responsibility in relation to safeguarding children.

Partnership working in children's services

The CAF is designed to be used by a range of agencies involved in the care of children and is a formal, standardised approach to the assessment of need. The aim is to promote earlier interventions and wellbeing. Government policy states that the child should be at the centre of care and that services – provided by integrated teams – should be working around the child.

Research summary: partnership working in services for children: use of the common assessment framework

Collins and McCray (2012) explored partnership in relation to the CAF, practitioners' understandings of their roles and partnership in education, health and social care contexts. Individual interviews were conducted with 20 practitioners from education, social care and health services. This sample included school nurses and health visitors.

Although they were using the common assessment framework, participants' practice was directed by targets that differed between services. There were also contradictions reported in terms of the requirement to enhance quality while reducing costs. Policy that is target-driven can detract from a holistic child-centred approach. The researchers concluded that practitioners experience challenges when working together within complex and dynamic practice and policy contexts.

Safeguarding vulnerable adults

The document *Safeguarding adults: the role of health service practitioners* states that *safeguarding adults is about the safety and well being of all patients but providing additional measures for those least able to protect themselves from harm or abuse* (DH, 2011a, p8).

Related activities range from prevention to multi-agency responses where harm and abuse occur. Empowering people to make their own decisions about their care is central to the policy. The local authority is the lead agency for safeguarding adults and coordinates the local Safeguarding Adults Board. Nurses are in a key position to identify a possible safeguarding concern – for example, when a vulnerable adult is admitted to hospital with unexplained injuries, or when a district nurse makes a home visit and suspects that family members may be abusing the patient (such abuse could be physical or psychological). In both cases local protocols and procedures will provide guidance on what should be done. Whatever the response is, it is likely to involve a range of professionals and agencies.

Research summary: partnership means protection? Perceptions of the effectiveness of multi-agency working and the regulatory framework within England and Wales

This research explored the effectiveness of the multi-agency approach and partnership working arrangements in adult protection. While examples of good practice were identified, there were also examples of insufficient sharing of information and lack of clarity regarding roles and responsibilities.
(Perkins et al., 2007)

Amid concerns for partnership working during the major programme of health service reforms, the government has clarified arrangements for safeguarding children and adults (NHS Commissioning Board, 2012a). Responsibility for safeguarding will sit in the Nursing Directorate of the DH, as part of the wider safety agenda. The NHS Commissioning Board and **Clinical Commissioning Groups** (CCGs) will have to ensure that the organisations from which they commission services have systems in place to safeguard children and vulnerable adults. Local authorities will continue to be the lead organisations for safeguarding. Local Safeguarding Children Boards and Safeguarding Adults Boards will continue their roles.

All NHS trusts have policies in place for reporting suspected abuse of children or vulnerable adults.

Activity 3.3   *Communication*

Think about a current or recent placement. What policies are in place for communicating suspected abuse of children or vulnerable adults?

---

continued . . .

Who is the designated lead professional for dealing with issues relating to safeguarding children and vulnerable adults?

There is a brief outline answer at the end of the chapter.

You will have found that recording all communication concerning suspected abuse is very important.

It appears from the examples and from research, cited above, that there is still work to do in relation to helping professionals to work collaboratively. 'Communities of practice' have been proposed as one way forward.

Communities of practice in interprofessional working

Concept summary: Community of Practice

Communities of practice (Wenger, 1998; **www.ewenger.com/theory/**) have been proposed as mechanisms to improve the quality of care. The focus of Wenger's theory is on learning as social participation and places learning in the context of *our lived experience of participation in the world* (Wenger, 1998, p3). A community of practice consists of a group of committed people who work collaboratively, learn together (the community) and through negotiation improve the quality of the care they provide (the practice). Quality enhancement is an incremental process and trust between the professionals is key to success.

Kilbride et al. (2011) report on the development of a community of practice in relation to stroke care.

Research summary: developing theory and practice

Kilbride et al. (2011) report on a case study that examined the processes involved in developing a new stroke unit. Action research was used to bring about changes in clinical practice and develop knowledge of the processes involved.

The findings revealed that building a team was important through joint working on projects that supported the work of the unit. A series of interprofessional seminars based on stroke guidelines helped staff transferred from disparate settings to the new unit to develop practice-based knowledge and skills in stroke care. Learning together became a strong theme. As the only group of professionals with round-the-clock presence on the unit, nurses were central to coordinating team activity. The appointment of a senior manager to support the developments helped to promote the profile of the unit within the hospital and externally. Through the focus on stroke care, individual professionals learned to work together, and as the success of the unit grew, staff felt part of something meaningful. Communities of practice are based on collegial relationships, with no room for hierarchical structures.

Kilbride et al.'s study suggests that there are benefits to interprofessional working, but time, effort and resources are needed in order to build effective interprofessional teams. The study suggests that by adopting the concept of 'community of practice' professionals can be helped to focus on their 'task' and thus overcome professional differences through learning together to enhance the quality of the care they provide.

Interprofessional working in end-of-life care

The DH (2008b) produced an 'end-of-life care strategy' based on best available research evidence, experience from hospices and examples of good practice. The DH adopts the following working definition of end-of-life care:

> *End of life care is care that:*
> *Helps all those with advanced, progressive, incurable illness to live as well as possible until they die. It enables the supportive and palliative care needs of both patient and family to be identified and met throughout the last phase of life and into bereavement. It includes management of pain and other symptoms and provision of psychological, social, spiritual and practical support.*
> (DH, 2008b, p47)

This definition implies interprofessional working, and the strategy states that care plans should be reviewed by a multidisciplinary team, patients and their carers. We will now return to Ivy's case study, which describes the last stage of her 'journey' when she was admitted to hospital in a very frail state. This stage of the case study involves a multidisciplinary team of healthcare professionals.

Case study: Ivy, Part 2

Over the next few years Ivy's physical condition gradually deteriorated as she became increasingly frail. She started to be reluctant to eat, but could usually be coaxed with her favourite foods. Following an overwhelming and debilitating urinary tract infection, Ivy was admitted to hospital in a very frail state. She was cared for in an acute medical ward, where she refused to get out of bed and refused to eat or drink, in spite of every effort

continued . . .

made by the nurses to encourage her. Her family also tried to tempt her with her favourite foods. Many discussions were held between various members of the healthcare team and Ivy's family concerning what to do about Ivy's refusal to eat or drink. The professionals involved in these discussions included the ward nurses, the consultant for elderly care, his registrar and senior house officer, and a gastro-enterologist. Ivy continued to resist any attempt at feeding. At one stage she said: You know what I want. *She pulled out naso-gastric tubes, and while feeding via a percutaneous enteral gastrostomy (PEG) was raised as a possibility, there were concerns about the safety of this approach. Eventually the difficult decision was made not to feed Ivy artificially. Ivy eventually passed away peacefully.*

In this case a difficult decision had to be made about whether or not to artificially feed Ivy. This represents a major ethical dilemma. First of all, the staff and family had to decide whether or not Ivy had the mental capacity to make a decision about her care and treatment. They used the 2005 Mental Capacity Act, which provides a framework to empower and protect adults who may lack the capacity to make some decisions for themselves. The act aims to provide a balance between an individual's rights to make their own decisions and their right to protection from harm if they lack such capacity. According to the act, every adult must be assumed to have capacity unless proved otherwise. You cannot assume someone lacks capacity on the basis of a diagnosis. Those in charge could not assume that Ivy lacked capacity just because she had been diagnosed with some form of dementia. Indeed, at one stage Ivy said to her carers: *You know what I want.* This statement, coupled with her repeated refusal to eat or drink and pulling out naso-gastric tubes, could be viewed as a statement that she did not want to be kept alive. However, no one could be certain that this was the case, as refusal to eat or drink is a symptom of late-stage dementia when patients forget what food is for, and forget what to do when food is placed in their mouths. Also, the act of pulling out naso-gastric tubes could have resulted from discomfort and/or confusion. This left the team of carers with a hugely difficult decision-making process as it was not possible to be sure whether Ivy's actions indicated that she did not wish to live any longer, or whether her actions were manifestations of her dementia. The Department for Constitutional Affairs (2007) produced a Code of Practice for the Mental Capacity Act. Guidance is provided on how to test if someone has mental capacity. The professional *directly concerned with the individual at the time the decision needs to be made* is the person who applies the test. As the proposed treatment for Ivy was the insertion of a PEG tube for feeding purposes, and Ivy would have needed to give consent for this to be performed, in this case the professional was the doctor. In order to assess mental capacity, it is necessary to determine if the individual can:

- understand the decision to be made;
- understand the consequences of making the decision, or not making the decision;
- understand, retain and use the information necessary to make the decision;
- communicate their decision.
(Department for Constitutional Affairs, 2007)

The outcome of this test applies to a particular decision. Each time a decision needs to be made, the test needs to be applied because sometimes patients can make some decisions but not others.

In Ivy's case the outcome of the test was that Ivy was not able to convey understanding of the decision concerning whether or not to receive artificial feeding. Consequently, in the absence of any other provision concerning Ivy's preferences, the team of carers had to make the decision on Ivy's behalf. Again, the Mental Capacity Act provides guidance in cases like this, advising that any decision made on behalf of the patient must be in their best interests, and any treatment option chosen must be the least restrictive one, that is, least restrictive of their basic rights and freedoms (Department for Constitutional Affairs, 2007).

Sometimes patients might not be in a position to make decisions for themselves, and it might be necessary to involve their families, significant others and carers. In this case, Ivy's family were central to the decision-making process in being able to provide background information about Ivy's life and the likelihood of her preferences in this situation. The Mental Capacity Act does provide for people to plan ahead for a time in the future when they might lack the capacity to make decisions – for example, through appointing a Power of Attorney or making a living will – but Ivy had not done this. There are frameworks designed to help decision-making in ethical situations such as this; they provide structure and bring objectivity to a process that, by its very nature, is emotional. Thompson et al.'s (2006) DECIDE framework provides the opportunity to work systematically through the decision-making process.

> **Concept summary: ethical decision-making – the DECIDE framework**
>
> **D**efine the problem
> **E**thical review
> **C**onsider options
> **I**nvestigate outcomes
> **D**ecide on action
> **E**valuate results
> (Thompson et al., 2006, pp322–4)

You can now think about how this framework might be used to involve Ivy's family in the decision-making process.

Activity 3.4   *Decision-making*

Bearing in mind the guidance provided by the Mental Capacity Act and the principles of decision-making outlined above, how would you, as Ivy's nurse, involve her family in this decision-making process?

What sort of information should they be given?

What is the role of the professional healthcare team?

There is a brief outline answer at the end of the chapter.

You will have noted the sensitive nature of this scenario and the need to support Ivy's family. The information that the family required would have included the treatment options, the advantages and disadvantages, the benefits and risks, and the likely outcomes. In short, they would need to be supplied with information about the evidence base for the insertion of PEG feeding tubes in patients like Ivy. Evidence suggests that the benefits of feeding patients with dementia with PEG tube are few (Sampson et al., 2009: Fenwick, 2010).

You will also have reassured Ivy's family that, although active treatment might not be pursued, nursing care would continue and every effort would be made to ensure Ivy's comfort and dignity were maintained. The role of the healthcare team is to provide information, to support the family and to protect Ivy from harm, ensuring that her best interests are guiding the process.

In this case the team decided that it was not in Ivy's best interests to insert a PEG tube, as there was insufficient evidence to support this intervention with patients like Ivy. They felt the tube would cause Ivy discomfort and she would be likely to try to pull it out, causing pain and complications. Her family believed that Ivy would not have wanted to be fed artificially and that she was reaching the end of her natural life. So, using the shared expertise of the healthcare team and the patient's family, the decision was made not to insert a PEG tube.

While Ivy and her family remained central to this decision-making process, the hospital team of professionals were also crucial in ensuring that Ivy's best interests were upheld.

Liverpool Care Pathway

The Liverpool Care Pathway for the Dying Patient (LCP) was not used in Ivy's case, but it is a tool that can be used in similar situations by multi-professional teams. The LCP was developed by the palliative care team at the Royal Liverpool and Broadgreen University Hospital NHS Trust and Marie Curie Cancer Care Hospice in Liverpool. The LCP is a multi-professional, evidence-based framework to guide care in the last days of life and has been identified as best practice in *Improving supportive and palliative care (CSGSP)* (NICE, 2004) and *End of life care strategy* (DH, 2008b). The tool is used when the multidisciplinary team agree that the patient is dying. Inappropriate interventions are stopped when the disadvantages outweigh the advantages (Ellershaw and Wilkinson, 2011; for more information about the LCP, go to the Marie Curie Palliative Care Institute Liverpool website at www.mcpcil.org.uk). However, while the LCP is widely used, it has attracted controversy in some national newspapers. For example, it was alleged in an article in *The Independent* (Harris, 2012) that the LCP is being used to hasten the deaths of terminally people – by withholding food and drink – to save resources.

Partnership working with individual patients

There are policies in place to assist partnership working with particular categories of patient – for example, Person Centred Planning for people with learning disabilities, the Care Programme Approach for people with mental health problems, the Single Assessment Process for older people. The Coalition government expects that shared decision-making will become the norm. Patients will have access to information necessary to make choices about their care, choice of any healthcare provider, consultant-led team, GP practice and treatment.

The Coalition government's vision for shared decision-making in healthcare entails patients and professionals working together in partnership to reach decisions about care and treatment. As government policy announcements do not always provide sufficient guidance on implementation, Coulter and Collins (2011) published a report that provides guidance on decision-making between individual patients and individual clinicians. They define shared decision-making as follows:

> *Shared decision-making is a process in which clinicians and patients work together to clarify treatment, management or self-management support goals, sharing information about opinions and preferred outcomes with the aim of reaching mutual agreement on the best course of action.*
> (Coulter and Collins, 2011, p2)

It is important to note that, aside from government policy, professional regulatory bodies expect clinicians to work in partnership with patients, informing and involving them whenever possible (Coulter and Collins, 2011, pvii). If patients are going to take part in making decisions about their care, they need to have information that is reliable, balanced and evidence-based. A patient's preferences must be recorded.

The process of shared decision-making entails sharing of experience and expertise. While the clinician brings expertise in diagnosis, pathophysiology, prognosis, treatment options and likelihood of outcomes to decision-making, the patient brings the lived experience of illness, socio-economic circumstances, values, beliefs and preferences (Coulter and Collins, 2011).

There are decision aids – for example, leaflets, computer programs, DVDs and interactive websites – for patients to use when decisions do not need to be made immediately. For information on some treatment options, patients can be directed to 'NHS Choices', an online service that provides information about the NHS and about health to help people to make choices about their health and healthcare (www.nhs.uk). However, such aids should not replace contact with clinicians. The information that patients require in order to reach informed decisions includes an account of the evidence base that supports treatment plans and any risks that might be attached to treatments, plus the benefits and risks attached to interventions.

Coulter and Collins (2011) suggest that shared decision-making is appropriate when decisions have to be made concerning whether to have a diagnostic test; receive medical, surgical or psychological interventions; take medication; or attempt a lifestyle change.

Case study: Sharon

Sharon is a 43-year-old woman who has had multiple sclerosis for 20 years. She is married and lives in a specially adapted bungalow with her husband and with her two children who are in their late teens. Sharon is now confined to a wheelchair as she is unable to walk, and she has limited use of her arms. She has a

continued . . .

permanent urinary catheter, and a district nurse visits Sharon regularly to change the catheter. Otherwise Sharon's care is provided by her immediate and extended family. Sharon has had increasingly frequent admissions to hospital. She was recently admitted to an acute medical ward of an NHS trust with a severe chest infection and is now very weak. She is also very anxious, as over the years she has developed her own routine for managing her multiple sclerosis, and during previous admissions to hospital this routine has become disrupted, which has caused her distress. Sharon is also becoming more dependent on her family and is worried about being a burden to them. She is wondering if it might be better for everyone if she moved into a care home, but she does not have much information about her eligibility for a place in a care home and she fears institutionalisation. Sharon's consultant is also wondering if her needs might be better met in a care home.

Activity 3.5   *Team working*

With the principles of 'no decision about me without me' and shared decision-making in mind, how do you think nurses can work in partnership with Sharon during her stay in hospital?

How can Sharon be helped to reach a decision about her future care?

There is a brief outline answer at the end of the chapter.

It is clear from the case study that Sharon's needs for care and support are increasing. However, moving into a care home is a major decision for her, and Sharon and her family need clear and balanced information before she makes a decision. Sharon must remain central to all discussions and decision-making. In such cases, counselling sometimes helps a patient to clarify their options and preferences. Often nurses are trained to undertake this role, which is sometimes referred to as 'health coaching' and helps people to develop the knowledge, skills and confidence necessary to make major decisions about their health, treatment and/or lifestyle changes (Coulter and Collins, 2011).

Chapter summary

This chapter has considered policies relating to working in partnership with individual patients, their families and carers, and with other professionals. Coulter and Collins (2011) suggest that patients who are involved in making decisions about their treatment tend to have better outcomes than those who are passive recipients of care and treatment. Interprofessional working is very much driven by the government, in the belief that it will enhance the quality of care. While there are small-scale studies that demonstrate some benefits of interprofessional working, overall the evidence is weak. Research does suggest that difficulties still exist as a result of professional differences and that in order for interprofessional working to be effective, the investment of time and resources might be *continued . . .* •••

necessary. In the next chapter, the theme of partnership working will continue, but in relation to groups rather than individual patients. Government policy concerning user involvement and public participation will also be explored.

Activities: Brief outline answers

Activity 3.1: Team working (page 46)

There are many possible answers. You might have chosen the WRVS, a voluntary organisation that runs hospital shops and cafés, welcome desks in hospitals and trolley rounds in wards. The organisation also 'befriends' people in hospital and in the community, and organises the Meals on Wheels service. Or you might have chosen an organisation dedicated to specific health problems, such as the British Heart Foundation, Diabetes UK and MIND.

Activity 3.2: Team working (page 48)

Your answer will depend on the nature of your placement. Inevitably, you will have identified working with doctors, and described reporting patients' responses to treatments, and their general progress, to doctors. Specifically, you might have identified a child with cystic fibrosis, in which case you might have described working closely with a physiotherapist in terms of timing the administration of medicines with physio-therapy treatments, and the positioning of patients.

Activity 3.3: Communication (pages 52–3)

Your answer will depend on the NHS trust you are working in. However, all trusts will have a designated lead for dealing with suspected abuse. The important point is that all communication must be recorded.

Activity 3.4: Decision-making (page 56)

First, the problem should be clearly defined with Ivy's family. They need to be given clear information about the options that are available, and the likely consequences of the various options, using an evidence base wherever possible. They need to be given time to think about the problem, possible actions and likely outcomes.

The role of the professional healthcare team is to be open and honest with Ivy's family, to respect their contribution to decision-making and to listen to their concerns and their beliefs about Ivy's likely preferences. The nurse should support Ivy's family throughout the process.

Activity 3.5: Team working (page 59)

The nurses caring for Sharon would make a detailed assessment of her, documenting her preferences for care and help with daily living activities, with the aim of adhering to Sharon's usual routines as far as possible. Sharon will need reliable information about the support that might be available to her at home and in a care home.

Further reading

Baggott, R (2007) *Understanding health policy.* Bristol: Policy Press.

Chapter 8, 'Partnerships and health policy', provides an excellent analysis of policy relating to partnership working in healthcare provision.

DH (2012) *End of life care strategy: fourth annual report.* London: DH.

This document contains tools to guide end-of-life care and case studies of good practice.

Goodman, B and Clemow, R (2010) *Nursing and collaborative practice: a guide to interprofessional learning and working* (2nd edn). Exeter: Learning Matters.

This book explores several aspects of interprofessional working and working in teams, with good application to nursing practice.

Griffith, R and Tengnah, C (2010) *Law and professional issues in nursing.* Exeter: Learning Matters.

This book considers legal, ethical and professional issues in nursing.

Grimshaw, K (2012) Safeguarding older patients. *Nursing Older People,* 24(7): 27–30.

This article describes the implementation of policy through case studies of older people.

Useful website

www.redcross.org.uk

The British Red Cross website provides information on the vital and wide ranging work that this voluntary organisation performs for society. For particular healthcare-related functions, select 'UK health and social care'.

Chapter 4
The policy context of patient and public involvement in healthcare

Chapter aims

After reading this chapter, you will be able to:

*   describe key policy developments in relation to service user involvement and public participation;
*   identify local initiatives/forums that engage with service users and the wider public;

- critically discuss the advantages and challenges of service user involvement and public participation;
- consider how nurses can make use of accounts of patient experiences to improve the quality of care.

Introduction

Scenario: Serena

Serena is a nurse working on a ward specialising in gastro-intestinal surgery. She is particularly impressed with the way some patients cope with surgery that results in the formation of a stoma. She has spent a lot of time listening to patients' accounts of their fears, their feelings about a change in body image, and the sort of interventions that have helped them to recover and develop a positive outlook. Serena is wondering how these rich accounts can be used to capture exactly what it is that helps patients to come to terms with their changed body image, so that the nurses can be clear about 'what works', and good practice can be clearly identified and used more explicitly to help all patients, but especially those who do not cope so well following surgery.

Serena talks to a senior staff nurse about her interest. The staff nurse is on a research course at the local university that provides education for the trust. She explains to Serena how government policy strongly encourages the use of patient experiences to improve the quality of care, as part of the wider patient and public involvement agenda. She also tells Serena that she has been learning how research approaches can be used to record patient stories. The staff nurse agrees with Serena that she will talk to one of the lecturers on the research course to explore how they can take this interest further.

In this chapter we consider the way policies urge us to focus on the patient experience and learn from patient feedback to improve the quality of care. Successive governments have wanted to address the 'democratic deficit' in healthcare through involving the wider public as well as service users. How does being a citizen, with a citizen's rights and responsibilities, include such public participation? We will look at developments since the 1990s to explore the way in which service user involvement has progressed and the different political motivations behind it, taking in various initiatives and forums that aim to address the democratic deficit. One policy aim of public participation/user involvement is to raise the quality of healthcare. You will consider areas where the public/health service users have been successful in influencing policy.

Definitions of terms

You will find various terms in the literature relating to patient and public involvement in healthcare. The term 'service user' is frequently used to refer to people who are receiving health and social services. On the other hand, 'public participation' refers to the wider involvement of members of society who are always 'potential' users of health and social services. More recently, the term 'patient and public involvement' has been adopted by central government.

Why should service users and the public be involved in healthcare decisions?

Activity 4.1   *Team working*

Why should service users and the public be consulted on the planning and delivery of healthcare services?

There is a brief outline answer at the end of the chapter.

In the activity, you might have thought about the value of patients' experiences in informing service development; you have already seen how Serena believed that nurses could learn from listening to patients' stories. As far as the wider public is concerned, the NHS is largely funded through general taxation and members of the public, as tax payers, have a right to comment on how their money is spent; furthermore, members of the public bring a perspective that is different from that of professionals (McIver, 1998).

Developments in public participation and user involvement

Public participation and user involvement in healthcare gained prominence during the 1990s. NHS patients have in the past been passive receivers of care, with little opportunity to exercise 'voice' in the planning of services or 'choice' in relation to treatment (North, 1977). They were expected to follow the advice of healthcare professionals; indeed, Klein (1984) described the NHS as *a monument to enlightened paternalism*. This approach has now changed, and individual patients are expected to have choice and be involved in decisions about their care and treatment, as we saw in Chapter 3. Furthermore, service user groups and the wider public are also invited to give their opinions on the planning and delivery of healthcare services. Reasons for this change in thinking include a perceived lack of democracy in healthcare services – often referred to as the 'democratic deficit' – and the continuing desire to improve the quality of healthcare.

During the 1970s measures were taken to improve accountability and patient representation in the NHS following several scandals in long-stay hospitals that raised serious questions about patients' interests (Baggott, 2004). In 1973, a Health Service Commissioner (also known as the **Ombudsman**) was appointed to investigate public complaints about maladministration, but the role of the Commissioner was not as extensive as it is now. In 1974, Community Health Councils were created in order to represent the views of the public, but their power was limited.

During the 1990s there was a concerted effort by the New Right governments to encourage users of health and social services to see themselves as consumers who, through enhanced awareness of their rights, would put pressure on local services to improve the quality of the care provided. At this time there was concern over the lack of choice that was available to health service users. In terms of the provision of both primary and secondary care, the NHS and Community Care Act in 1990 required health authorities to involve local people in the planning and delivery of services. Health authorities were required to involve local people in the assessments of their needs; social service departments were required to consult users, carers and voluntary organisations during the production of community care plans. In particular, the policy document *Local voices* (NHSME, 1992) urged health authorities to consult users in planning and monitoring services to try to make services more responsive to local needs. This period saw the beginning of consultation with the public, using methods such as postal surveys, opinion polls, focus groups and community panels.

In 1995, Cooper et al. acknowledged that health authorities had employed several methods to engage with the public, but argued that the initiatives tended to consult the public rather than enable it to participate more actively in decision-making. They claimed that there was little shared understanding of the public's dual role as consumer and citizen.

> **Concept summary: models of user involvement**
>
> Drawing on the experience of user involvement in social work, Barnes and Walker (1996) describe two models of user involvement.
>
> - The consumerist model, which offers users a choice between products.
> - The empowerment model, which involves users in the development and delivery of services.

It has become evident that involving users in the development and delivery of health services is not necessarily an easy process and requires resources. Beresford and Croft (1993) identified the need for resources such as time, space, skill, and support and information. Training is needed for both service users and professionals as new values and skills are required for partnership working. It is essential to the process that there is equality of opportunity and access, and there must also be forums that facilitate involvement.

In 1996, the NHS Executive published guidance on patient and public involvement in decision-making in the NHS in the document *Patient partnership: building a collaborative strategy*. The guidance included providing information to service users, assisting service users to develop the requisite skills for partnership working, and supporting staff in partnership working. It was obviously a way of working that did not come naturally and needed some impetus.

These requirements to actively engage with services users and the public came at a time of extensive change in the NHS. Neither the health authorities nor patients were accustomed to the change in relationship that was required for such engagement to take place. Traditionally, professionals made the decisions, and generally patients were deferential towards professionals. Greenwell (1996) argued that regarding the patient as an equal partner in healthcare represented a radical departure from the traditional approach to provision of healthcare. There was also an assumption that patients and the public were willing and able to become involved in decision-making in a meaningful way, and accept the responsibility for such activity.

Does the public want to be involved?

Litva et al. (2002) investigated the extent of willingness of members of the public to engage in decision-making. The research presents a mixed picture of public willingness to become involved, with many participants expressing a desire for public opinion to be taken into account, and with some fearing that members of the public might be too subjective in their assessments.

Research summary: 'The public is too subjective': public involvement at different levels of healthcare decision-making

The background to this research was the requirement to elicit public views on decision-making in healthcare. The researchers used focus groups and in-depth interviews with members of the public, drawn from electoral rolls, pre-existing health-related organisations and pre-existing non-health-related organisations.

Decisions to be made at three levels were chosen.

- At health system level: the health authority can provide emergency services in one specialist centre or more basic treatment in two hospitals.
- At programme level: the health authority can fund either a new cancer ward or a new mental health ward.
- At individual level: two patients require expensive and effective drug treatment but the health authority can only fund one patient.

In each case the research participants were asked if they would like the public to be involved in making decisions about how the health authority should use its funds and how the funds should be allocated.

The findings revealed variations in the willingness of members of the public to engage in healthcare decision-making. While there was willingness for the public to be involved at system and programme levels, this was much less the case at the level of individual patients. The participants believed that health professionals should be responsible for these decisions. The research participants favoured consultation at system and programme levels and did not want to be held responsible for decisions that were made. The participants did not want to be involved in making decisions relating to treatments for individual patients.

(Litva et al., 2002)

So, while members of the public appreciated being informed and consulted on healthcare service development in line with the approach of the consumerist model, they were more reluctant to engage in an empowerment model approach.

Citizenship

Successive government policies have emphasised the role of the consumer, but also reflected renewed concern with issues of citizenship. From 1945 to the early 1970s, the goals of welfare provision were broadly accepted by the main political parties. However, by the 1990s, against the background of increasing demand for welfare services, coupled with a desire to reduce public expenditure, the series of New Right governments (1979–1997) sought to redefine the boundaries of the welfare state. New Right governments argued that the welfare state reduced individuals' capacity to care for themselves and their families as they became increasingly dependent on the state for benefits and welfare services. Thus there were attempts to reduce the number of people who were dependent on the state for services and support, and to increase the role of the voluntary and private sectors. This amounted to a move away from universal provision to a more selective provision – to those with the greatest need – as the governments aimed for a reduced role for the state in the provision of welfare services. These changes forged a change in the relationship between the individual and the state, often discussed within the context of citizenship.

Concept summary: citizenship

While citizenship is a contested concept and has attracted various definitions, there is agreement among many authors that the concept of citizenship concerns the relationship between the individual and the state. Conceptions of citizenship fall into three broad categories.

*   Formal citizenship relates to nationality and formal membership of a state, which confers rights and responsibilities.
*   Substantive citizenship concerns social rights; according to Steenbergen (1994), social rights are meant to give the formal status of citizenship a material foundation.
*   Citizenship as a sense of belonging involves engagement in public life through participation in the community.

In a seminal and influential essay, Marshall (1964) described the rights that were conferred on British citizens as the welfare state evolved, and that give substance to formal citizenship. The essay addresses Marshall's conceptualisation of society's move towards equality that began in the eighteenth century and culminated in the egalitarian policies of twentieth-century Britain. Marshall describes three elements of citizenship.

*   Civil rights developed in the eighteenth century and involve the rights necessary for individual freedom – for example, freedom of speech and religion, the right to justice and the right to equal justice in law.

- Political rights developed in the nineteenth century and concern the right to participate in the exercise of political power, either by exercising the right to vote or by standing for political office.
- Social rights involve: *the whole range from the right to a modicum of economic welfare and security to the right to share to the full in the social heritage and to live the life of a civilised being according to the standards prevailing in the society* (Marshall, 1964, p74).

The provisions of the post-war welfare state – for example, education, social security and healthcare – were perceived as having an equalising effect on individuals through the reduction in risk and insecurity. It could be argued that they strengthened a sense of community. Citizenship can, therefore, be seen both as a status and as a set of rights that arise as a consequence of this status (Barbalet, 1988). Prior et al. (1995) refer to citizenship as a concept of *being* and *doing* – citizenship being a status that people possess and a practice in which people engage.

This notion of citizenship as entailing activity was employed by the New Right governments through the promotion of 'active citizenship', which entails citizens taking some responsibility for some of the needs of society, rather than expecting the state to do everything (Oliver, 1993). Examples include voluntary organisations, charities and neighbourhood watch schemes. Further, the active citizen was expected to become involved in calling health services to account. Participation in public life is therefore seen as both a right and a duty of citizenship.

User involvement

When New Labour came to power in 1997 the emphasis on user involvement continued but with different philosophical underpinnings: there was an emphasis on active citizenship within a moral community. This was embraced through a new contract between the citizen and the state, with rights matched by responsibilities (DH, 1997). New Labour adopted 'third way' politics as a framework for policy-making. The 'third way' is somewhere between old-style **social democracy** and **neo-liberalism** (Giddens, 1998) and involves devolution, the renewal of the public sphere, more direct democracy and *no rights without responsibilities*.

The concept of user and public involvement was central to many of the policies introduced by the White Paper *The new NHS: modern, dependable* (DH, 1997). A series of policy documents ensured that user and public involvement was high on the NHS agenda at all levels. *A first class service* (DH, 1998a) claimed that the active participation of professionals and patients throughout the NHS was needed. The vision of the *NHS Plan* (DH, 2000a) included a health service *designed around the patient* (p10). The plan required each health authority to establish an independent local advisory forum made up of local residents to provide a sounding board for determining health priorities and policies. Lay membership of all the professional regulatory bodies was increased. *Shifting the balance of power* (DH, 2001b) set out the government's proposals to shift power and resources to frontline staff, service users and taxpayers. *Involving patients and the public in healthcare: a discussion document* (DH, 2001c) set out proposals for implementing the vision of a patient-centred NHS outlined in the NHS Plan: the voices of patients, their carers and the public were to be heard and listened to at every level of the NHS. The 2001 Health and Social Care Act made it a duty for the NHS to involve the public in the planning and development of services and in major decisions. All these developments were driven by concern about the governance of public services.

It is clear from the above that a concerted effort by the New Labour governments firmly placed user and public involvement at the heart of the NHS, and had a strong desire to move from a consumerist approach to a more empowering approach. New Labour went on to establish organisations such as:

- a national commission for patient and public involvement;
- patient advocacy and liaison services (PALS);
- patients' forums;
- local authority overview and scrutiny committees.

Patient Advice and Liaison Services (PALS)

PALS were introduced to ensure that the NHS listens to patients, their relatives and carers when they are using the NHS. The service attempts to help with addressing concerns as soon as possible and provides information, including how to make a complaint. The service is available in every NHS Trust and should be easily recognisable and accessible to patients.

Activity 4.2   *Communication*

Locate the PALS desk in your NHS Trust. What sort of work are they doing?

For further information on PALS, visit the website: www.pals.nhs.uk.

There is a brief outline answer at the end of the chapter.

Local Involvement Networks (LINks)

LINks are found in every geographical area. They are independent organisations consisting of networks of individuals and community groups who wish to become involved in improving the quality of local health and social care services. LINks give information to the commissioners and providers of health and social care services on the experiences and opinions of local people. If there is a particular health or social care issue that the local population feels needs to be addressed, then LINks will take this up on their behalf. LINks can ask health and social care providers for information, and the provider has a duty to respond. LINks can also carry out visits to local services, and if anything untoward is found, they can refer issues to the local Overview and Scrutiny Committee.

Overview and Scrutiny Committees

Overview and Scrutiny Committees are located in local government; they are made up of councillors, who are locally elected. Health Overview and Scrutiny Committees were established by the 2001 Health and Social Care Act in order to monitor local health services and ensure that these services are in the best interests of the local population. Overview and Scrutiny Committees have statutory powers and can make recommendations to local NHS bodies, and the NHS has to consult the committee when developing services.

Degrees of involvement

A frequently cited 'ladder' of citizen participation was published by Arnstein (1969). Activities are grouped hierarchically and range from *degrees of citizen power*, e.g. citizen control and partnership to *non-participation*, e.g. therapy and manipulation. As initiatives progress up the ladder towards citizen control, they become increasingly empowering. Arguably, however, many initiatives are still functioning around the level of consultation.

Consultation

There has been a desire to learn from the patient experience for some time – this has been expressed through the patient satisfaction surveys. Since 2007 every acute NHS trust has been required to take part in the Patient Survey Programme in order to elicit patients' views and use this information to improve the quality of care. Since 2009 the Patient Reported Outcome Measures (PROMs) (DH, 2008c) programme requires NHS trusts to collect and record self-reported measures of health before and after specific elective interventions: hip and knee replacement surgery, hernia repair and varicose vein surgery. There are plans to extend the range of conditions covered by PROMs to include mental health, cancer care, asthma, chronic obstructive pulmonary disease, diabetes, epilepsy, heart failure and stroke (Barham and Devlin, 2011). The aim is to focus on outcomes of interventions, and the uses of the data collected include informing patient choice and measuring and rewarding performance. Barham and Devlin (2011) stress the relevance of PROMs for nursing, and point out that the use of PROMs by nurses provides them with an opportunity to develop the evidence base for nursing practice.

Activity 4.3	*Evidence-based practice and research*

What measures are in place in your clinical placement, or at NHS trust level, to gain the views of the patients on their experiences of care and treatment?

There is a brief outline answer at the end of the chapter.

Government policy aims for patients and the public to have more input to informing decisions about the commissioning of services. The placement or NHS trust might make use of patient surveys and satisfaction questionnaires. However, surveys and questionnaires are often designed by service providers and ask questions from the service point of view. These can elicit information that the service wants, but that information is not necessarily what the service user wants to tell the service provider. Individual patient experiences can be used for such purposes. Lees (2011) supports the use of patient stories, gathered through narrative-based forms of inquiry, to learn from patients and to gain greater understanding of the patient's experience.

While members of the public may sometimes be reticent, some service user groups have been highly successful and provide opportunities to inform policy as well as service development. While the use of surveys can provide useful information, they do tend to operate at the level of consultation. Other initiatives – for example, the Expert Patients programme – use a more collaborative approach.

Collaboration

Expert Patients

Expert Patient policy evolved in the late 1990s in response to the growing number of people with long-term illnesses such as diabetes. Clinicians realised they had underestimated the contribution the patient can make to the management of these illnesses because of what they know through personal experience.

Wilson (2001) describes the Expert Patient initiative as an example of the active participation of patients as experts and partners in care. The concept originated at Stanford University, California, USA, when Professor Kate Lorig developed programmes for people with arthritis using trained lay leaders as educators. Originally called the Chronic Disease Self Management model, the programmes equipped people with arthritis with the skills to manage their own condition, with much success (Donaldson, 2003).

Wilson (2001) questions whether the term 'expert' can truly be applied to a patient in the same sense as to a professional, suggesting that 'expertise' is usually acquired through education. In the policy context of the expert patient (DH, 2001d), the definition of expert appears to assume that the expertise is derived from experience, not education (Wilson, 2001).

Fears have been expressed that the management of long-term conditions could become too much of a personal responsibility, with a reduction in state responsibility (Wilson, 2001), though Expert Patient programmes should not always been seen as cost-cutting measures, as there is always the possibility that empowered patients might make more demands on resources as their knowledge increases. However, Wilson cites the benefits of Expert Patient programmes in the UK such as improved wellbeing and a reduction in demand on health service resources.

User groups

There is some evidence of success for user groups in developing specific healthcare services. *The NHS cancer plan* (DH, 2000c) charged cancer networks with taking account of the views of patients and carers when planning services. Richardson et al. (2005) investigated the achievements of cancer partnership groups.

> **Research summary: 'Working the system': achieving change through partnership working: an evaluation of cancer partnership groups**
>
> The research investigated the characteristics and achievements of cancer partnership groups – collaborative service improvement groups formed of NHS staff and service users. The research used a telephone survey, face-to-face interviews and document analysis. The research found that cancer partnership groups engaged in a range of activities from initiatives to improve the patient experience – for example, information leaflets – to the work of well-established groups that were able to influence new service developments (Richardson et al., 2005).

Control

While user involvement is government driven and thus a 'top-down' approach (Barnes, 1999), there have been examples of 'bottom-up' movements by groups of people who were dissatisfied with the services they were receiving, and there are some examples of areas where service users have taken greater control, such as in mental health services and in the disability movement.

> ### Case study: the disability movement
>
> *The British Council of Organisations of Disabled People (BCODP) was formed in 1981 in response to dissatisfaction with statutory services and voluntary organisations that were led by able-bodied people. A distinction is drawn between organisations of disabled people and those for disabled people. The BCODP adopted a social model of disability, identifying the barriers that are imposed on disabled people by society. The emphasis is on agency, and the BCODP has successfully campaigned against discrimination, and for disabled people's rights. The organisation is now called the UK Disabled People's Council and is an umbrella body for disabled people's organisations in the UK (www.ukdpc.net).*

Further measures to increase control have entailed extending choice over welfare services, for example, through direct payments and personal budgets, which have met with some success for some client groups, particularly people with disabilities.

Personal health budgets

Drawing on some of the successes with direct payments and personal budgets for support from social services, Lord Darzi proposed the introduction of personal health budgets in his *NHS next stage review* (DH, 2008a). The initiative was to be part of the plan to personalise the NHS and make it more responsive to patients, giving individuals more control over their lives. The Coalition government confirmed its support for continuing personal health budgets in the White Paper *Equity and excellence. liberating the NHS* (DH, 2010a).

A leaflet designed for patients states: *Personal health budgets offer the opportunity to work in equal partnership with the NHS about how your health and wellbeing needs can best be met. They are one way to have choice and control of your healthcare and support* (DH, 2012d, p2).

Personal health budgets are intended for people with long-term conditions and represent a sum of money to support individual healthcare and wellbeing needs – they exclude primary and emergency care. Anyone who is eligible for a personal health budget will engage in an assessment of needs, and the person will then be told how much money is available to them. A planning process with the local NHS team follows, and the resulting plan is presented to a panel by the local personal health budget lead. Once the budget is agreed, the plan is signed off by the relevant PCT.

The money can be provided as:

- a notional budget, which means that spending the money is planned and agreed with the local NHS team, which arranges the care and support on behalf of the individual patient.
- a real budget held by a third party that helps the individual to decide what their needs are, and, in agreement with the local NHS team, organises and buys the care and support on behalf of the patient.

The payment of money directly to individual patients has to be piloted. The acceptance of a personal health budget is not obligatory, and if people with long-term conditions feel that their current arrangements meet their needs, then those arrangements will not change. Personal health budgets have been piloted with mental health service users and people with long-term conditions. The type of services they have bought include therapies, personal care, respite, equipment and self-management courses (DH, 2012d).

Research summary: personal health budgets

Davidson et al. (2012) present an interim report on experiences and outcomes for personal health budget holders. Fifty-two people with long-term conditions were interviewed nine months after being offered a personal health budget; they were drawn from 17 PCTs involved in the pilot of personal health budgets in England. Thirteen carers of budget holders were also interviewed.

The findings revealed the potential for personal health budgets to lead to improvements in health and wellbeing. Most interviewees said that personal health budgets had improved their health. People with long-term physical health problems also reported improvements in their mental health and vice versa. People with mental health problems experienced less stress, reduced use of emergency services and better management of relapses. Patients and carers appreciated greater choice and control over aspects of healthcare, and increased flexibility and access to goods and services not provided by the NHS, e.g. exercise classes, gym membership, complementary therapies. Furthermore, the majority felt comfortable making choices, though those who were employing carers and personal assistants them-selves expressed the need for information and support. However, a minority experienced difficulties understanding the budget and how to use it. PCT management sometimes resulted in delays in procuring services. Some people were also receiving social care funding, and there were some reports of lack of clarity about social care and healthcare responsibilities and what could be funded from each budget.

User involvement: product and process

The aim of user involvement is to improve the quality of health services and make them more responsive to the needs of the local population: the product. However, the process of becoming involved can also have benefits for individuals as they engage with fellow users, often learn more about their health problems, and sometimes gain confidence and enhanced self-esteem.

Case study: service user involvement in mental health services

Vivienne is a 42-year-old woman who has suffered with mental health problems for 10 years. She takes medication and is admitted to hospital from time to time when her problems become acute and she feels she is not coping. As a long-time user of mental health services, Vivienne was invited to join her local mental health user group. At first she was not at all sure, but decided to 'give it a go'. Through meeting fellow services users Vivienne made some new friends, but also improved her own understanding of her health problem by sharing her experiences with others and listening to other users' stories. Vivienne gradually grew in strength as she felt better able to cope with her condition and take more control over her life. As she became more empowered, she no longer felt a victim of her health problem. Vivienne's confidence and skills have improved to the extent that she now engages with fellow users in advising the local providers on the delivery of local mental health services, and she also talks to student nurses at the local university education centre. This process has been described by Dalrymple and Burke (1995) as one of sharing biography, changed consciousness and political action.

Activity 4.4   *Communication*

Are there any service user groups operating in your area of practice?

If you are not aware of any, at some time during your nursing education you will experience service users contributing to lessons. What can you learn from this?

Where do you think service user involvement can be most successful?

There is a brief outline answer at the end of the chapter.

Service user involvement groups have often centred on a particular aspect of care, but attention has turned to involvement in **care pathways** where continuity of care is essential. The following two research summaries illustrate this.

Research summary: user involvement in stroke services

The study (Jones et al., 2008) used action research to involve users of local stroke services in service development. It was driven by a perceived need to go beyond consultation and to engage patients and carers in the service development agenda. The findings revealed that service users can play a meaningful role in planning services. The research also found that from the perspective of patients and carers, the provision of information, preparation for transfer of care and the integration of social and leisure activities were the priorities for service development. The findings were used to inform the development of the local stroke pathway.

Research summary: service user involvement in integrated care pathways

The research aimed to explore the possibilities for involving users in the development of the NHS in England through integrated care pathways (ICPs). Smith and Ross (2007) undertook a systematic literature review relating to user involvement in ICPs for cataract care, hip replacement and knee arthroscopy. The findings relate to the use of patients' views and experiences for service development and planning, and improving the delivery of services. While there was general satisfaction with the services received, Smith and Ross suggest that more work needs to be done in relation to patients' expectations and needs, the development of ICPs that are sufficiently structured to maximise outcomes but remain flexible enough to cater for individuals' diverse needs, and methods for integrating patients' experiences into service development.

Professional and management responses to service user involvement initiatives

Management responses to service user involvement initiatives have been mixed. There appears to be tension between the statutory duty to engage with service users and the requirement for professionals and managers to exercise their responsibility in relation to the provision of services. The following is an example.

Scenario: a long-stay ward for older people

Beverley is a manager of a ward for older people in a local community hospital. The hospital provides short-stay care for people with long-term conditions, and people who need rehabilitation. Some patients use the service regularly to provide respite for their carers, and to prevent their condition from deteriorating to a stage where they

continued . . .

require admission to an acute NHS trust. The service acts as a 'bridge' between hospital and home. The ward has an established user group made up of patient representatives and their families.

The user group has requested that family pets be allowed on to the ward so that patients can maintain contact with their pets, and the ward can feel more homely. Beverley is duty bound to listen to the user group and to attempt to meet their needs. However, she also has a professional responsibility for the safety of her patients, and has to consider whether all patients would be comfortable with pets on the ward. Some patients might have fears, and/or allergies to certain pets. She also has to consider what sorts of pets families might want to bring on to the ward. There is a lot for her to consider, and consult on, before she can engage in further discussion with the user group.

In the early days of user involvement researchers found that managers and professionals liked the idea but wanted to remain in control of determining policy (Milewa et al., 1998, 1999; Harrison and Mort, 1998). Milewa et al. reported that health authority managers adhered to their own professional and statutory responsibility for planning health services. Harrison and Mort reported that there was a tendency for managers to question the legitimacy of user groups, particularly in relation to the extent to which members of user groups represented, or did not represent, the wider community.

The Coalition government, and patient and public participation

The series of Labour governments (1997–2010) pursued an agenda of devolved power to local levels and encouraged people to be more active in their communities. This has continued with the Coalition government through their **Big Society** agenda. However, while the local agenda may remain similar, there are differences in the political views behind the agenda. While New Labour viewed central government as supporting and enabling local engagement and participation, the Coalition government views central government as preventing local activity and community engagement (Brodie et al., 2011). The Coalition government has also made severe cuts in public spending, which can have the effect of reducing local participation if local groups and organisations lose their funding.

Nevertheless, the Coalition government has committed to strengthening patient and public involvement (DH, 2010a). There is a certain degree of continuity of policy, though the government has created a *powerful new consumer champion* in **Healthwatch England**, which is located in the Care Quality Commission. Healthwatch England receives information from local Healthwatch organisations that is used to provide advice to the NHS Commissioning Board, Monitor (the economic regulator) and the Secretary of State (DH, 2010a). HealthWatch England will provide leadership, advice and support to local Healthwatch services when these take over from LINks in April 2013. Local Healthwatch organisations will continue, and build on, the work of LINks, ensuring that the views of local people are used to inform commissioning of health and social care services. They will be funded by, and accountable to, local authorities.

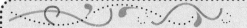

Chapter summary

This chapter has traced developments in service user involvement and public participation from earlier initiatives that were based on consulting people to more complex initiatives that engage people more meaningfully in planning service provision. Listening to the voices of patients, their carers and the wider public remains high on the government's agenda. This agenda is informed by a desire to use the views of service users to enhance the quality of care and to make that care more responsive to the needs of local populations. Nurses engage in this policy when they seek feedback from their patients, and the information gained can be used to develop their practice.

Activities: Brief outline answers

Activity 4.1: Team working (page 64)

Patients can make valuable contributions to the planning and delivery of healthcare services because of their personal experiences of living with illness, and of being receivers of healthcare services. The public know their communities well and are in a good position to comment on their needs.

Activity 4.2: Communication (page 69)

The work of PALS includes: providing patients with information about the NHS; listening to the concerns of patients and their families about the NHS; trying to resolve concerns that people have when using the NHS; providing information about complaints procedures; and providing an early warning system for NHS trusts by alerting them to problems.

Activity 4.3: Evidence-based practice and research (page 70)

Patient surveys and satisfaction surveys are in widespread use.

Activity 4.4: Communication (page 74)

Your answer will depend on your area of practice or placement. For example, user groups are well established within mental health services, with service users being involved in discussions about service development, contributing to teaching students and often sitting on panels to interview new staff.

It is likely that you will have experience of service users participating in teaching sessions, and you will probably have acknowledged the value of hearing about their experiences of care and treatment.

Further reading

Bach, S and Ellis, P (2011) *Leadership, management and team working*. Exeter: Learning Matters.

This book addresses the challenges of working in teams, conflict management, negotiation and managing change.

Beresford, P (2005) Service user: regressive or liberatory terminology? *Disability & Society*, 20(4): 469–77.

This book offers a critical discussion of the term 'service user' with a particular focus on disabled people.

Lees, C (2011) Measuring the patient experience. *Nurse Researcher*, 19(1): 25–8.

This article contains an excellent discussion concerning the use of surveys and patient stories to improve quality of care.

Nicol, J (2011) *Nursing adults with long-term conditions*. Exeter: Learning Matters.

This book equips nurses with the knowledge and skills required to care for people with long-term conditions.

Reed, A (2011) *Nursing in participation with patients and carers*. Exeter: Learning Matters.

This book explores nurse–patient relationships, and discusses how quality of patient experiences can be assessed.

Useful website

www.networks.nhs.uk

This website provides practical guides to patient and public involvement in healthcare services.

Chapter 5
The policy context of trust and public safety

continued . . .

By entry to the register:

xiv. Works within policies to protect self and others in all care settings including in the home care setting.

Chapter aims

After reading this chapter, you will be able to:

- outline key policies concerning patient safety;
- identify latent and active errors in patient case studies;
- discuss policy relating to caring for people with learning disabilities;
- describe the features of good practice in relation to the implementation of policy concerning patient safety;
- critically discuss why patients may lack trust in healthcare systems.

Introduction

In this chapter we will explore aspects of patient safety, and you will consider stories of the care received by some patients with learning disabilities (MENCAP, 2007) in order to appreciate how failure to adhere to relevant policies can compromise a patient's safety.

Patient safety is high on the health policy agenda, and this chapter will use relevant literature to explore how, through human error and increasingly complex healthcare systems, **latent conditions** allow **active failures** to happen. Patient safety has attracted attention at international levels (WHO, USA, EU) as well as at national and local policy levels. The work of the National Patient Safety Agency (NPSA) will be included, and you will consider failures in care and relate them to practice. We will look at examples of good nursing practice in relation to implementing policy concerning safety. Media coverage of failures in patient safety has contributed to concerns about trust in healthcare systems. A case study of refugees and asylum seekers will be used in this chapter to explore aspects of trust in healthcare professionals and healthcare systems, because patient diversity means we need to consider the particular needs of patients from different backgrounds in building trusting relationships.

Policy on patient safety

Patient safety is *the process by which an organisation makes patient care safer* (Bird and Dennis, 2005, p52).

The NPSA defines a patient safety incident as:

> *any unintended or unexpected incident which could have or did lead to harm for one or more patients receiving NHS-funded care. This is also referred to as an adverse event/incident or clinical error, and includes near misses.* (NPSA, 2004)

Examples of patient safety incidents include medication errors, unclear documentation, equipment failure, incorrect advice and misdiagnosis (Woodward, 2006).

Two important key documents – *To err is human* (Kohn et al., 2000) from the USA and *An organisation with a memory* (DH, 2000b) from the UK – prompted global attention on patient safety (DH, 2006b). Both documents acknowledge that human beings make errors, but they also argue that errors can be prevented by designing systems that make it more difficult for people to do the wrong thing. With increasing complexity in healthcare delivery, the potential for errors expands (DH, 2000b; Kohn et al., 2000; DH, 2006b). It is estimated that 1 in 10 patients admitted to hospitals in developed countries will be unintentionally the victim of an error: around 50 per cent of these events could have been avoided if lessons had been learned from previous incidents. The same errors and system failures are often repeated (DH, 2006b). As well as failure to learn from incidents, these figures suggest that there are likely to be other contributory factors we have yet to explore.

International policy

In 2002, the WHO urged member states to strive to improve patient safety and the quality of care. In 2004, the World Alliance on Patient Safety was created (WHO, 2012). In setting up this alliance, the WHO recognised the complexity of the context of modern healthcare, which is characterised by rapid developments in technology and staff working under pressure, raising the potential for harm to patients. The alliance aimed to raise awareness of patient safety issues and to seek global solutions. It is now called WHO Patient Safety, and it leads a programme of international collaboration on patient safety and the dissemination of good practice.

Patient safety has attracted further attention at European Union level.

*   The Luxembourg Declaration on Patient Safety (European Commission, 2005) recommended a collaborative approach between health professionals and healthcare providers in order to enhance patient safety; the implementation of projects on patient safety in the workplace; ensuring that patients and their relatives are aware of **near misses** and **adverse events**.
*   The Council of the European Union recommendation on patient safety, including the prevention and control of healthcare-associated infections (Council of the European Union, 2009), included the proposal that patient safety be embedded as a priority issue in health policies and programmes at national, regional and local levels. Emphasis was also placed on the inclusion of patient safety in undergraduate and postgraduate education, and continuing professional development for health professionals.

National policy

Maximising patient safety is an essential component of the wider quality improvement agenda (Car et al., 2008, p73). It is not surprising, then, that a lot of attention has been paid to safety in recent health policy, and international policy aims can be traced in UK health policy. Soon after taking up the post of Health Secretary, Andrew Lansley challenged the NHS to put patient safety first (DH, 2010c). This emphasis on safety represents a continuation of the driving force behind the quality agenda set out in Lord Darzi's report:

Continuously improving patient safety should be at the top of the healthcare agenda for the 21st century. The injunction to 'do no harm' is one of the defining principles of the clinical professions . . . Public trust in the NHS is conditional on our ability to keep patients safe when they are in our care.
(DH, 2008a, p44)

Several initiatives had been set up by the Labour government.

- The NPSA was created in 2001 with the aim of improving the safety of patients in NHS-funded care in England and Wales. The agency collects data concerning patient safety, monitors adverse events, and provides guidance on patient safety (Milligan and Dennis, 2004). The safety functions of the NPSA will transfer to the NHS Commissioning Board as part of the NHS reforms.
- The National Reporting and Learning System (NRLS), created in 2004 within the NPSA, is a reporting system for patient safety incidents and near-miss events. Analysis of this information allows for trends to be identified and for advice to be disseminated (Bird, 2005). The NRLS will transfer to Imperial College Healthcare NHS Trust as part of the NHS reforms.

National policy initiatives have to be implemented locally. We will now look at selected policy documents and how they inform local policy.

Local policy

When mistakes are made, it is usually because of human error combined with organisational factors. In 2006, the Department of Health issued a report *Safety First: a report for patients, clinicians and healthcare managers* (DH, 2006b) in which it is stressed that the everyday experience of patients will reflect the extent to which a healthcare system is addressing the safety agenda. The document also calls for managers to make safety a priority and to support staff in implementing safer practices. The following scenario provides an example of peer pressure on junior staff to deviate from safety procedures in order to cope with a heavy workload.

Scenario: Joseph

Joseph is a third-year student nurse on a placement on an acute medical ward. His mentor is away on a study day, and he is working with a bank nurse who is not familiar with the ward. Joseph and the bank nurse have a group of patients to care for who are very dependent. Joseph is working hard to assess and prioritise the needs of these patients. The bank nurse gives Joseph a medicine cup with two tablets in it and tells him to give them to Mrs Andrews and then help her to get another patient out of bed. Joseph explains to the bank nurse that Mrs Andrews needs a lot of encouragement and help to take her tablets so he will not be able to help her immediately. The bank nurse tells him to leave the tablets on Mrs Andrews' locker as she needs help with her patient now.

Joseph feels quite pressured by the requests of the bank nurse, but he is clear that he cannot do what he is being asked to do, and tells this to the nurse. First, he tells her that he cannot administer the medication as he has not

continued . . .

been involved in checking the package it came from with Mrs Andrews' prescription chart. Second, he tells her that he cannot leave the tablets on Mrs Andrews' locker as anyone could take them, and even if Mrs Andrews did take the tablets herself, it would not be possible to record the time at which she took them – this could have implications for the timing of administration of further medication later. Third, Joseph explains to the nurse that if Mrs Andrews needs the tablets now, then he must be allowed to take his time to help her to swallow the tablets now; if medications are not administered at the prescribed time, this can constitute an error.

The bank nurse is not happy with Joseph's response, but she knows he is right and apologises to him, explaining that she is feeling under pressure herself with the heavy workload and lack of familiarity with the ward. Joseph feels pleased that he has resisted the pressure to engage in unsafe practice.

In 2004, the NPSA published the good practice guide *Seven steps to patient safety: an overview guide for NHS staff.* These are the seven steps.

1. Build a safety culture.
2. Lead and support your staff.
3. Integrate your risk management activity.
4. Promote reporting.
5. Involve and communicate with patients and the public.
6. Learn and share safety lessons.
7. Implement solutions to prevent harm.

Activity 5.1   *Leadership and management*

Think about a recent or current clinical placement. What measures can you identify within that placement to promote the safety of patients? For example, can you locate and describe the policy for reporting incidents? Are you aware of any patient safety champions within the department? What risk assessments take place?

There is a brief outline answer at the end of the chapter.

In 2009, the Healthcare Commission published its report *Safely does it: implementing safer care for patients.* (The Healthcare Commission's work in England has since been taken over by the Care Quality Commission.) The document reported on an investigation of how organisations were implementing safer care in three areas of recognised risk to patient safety: inpatient falls; implementation of actions required in safety alerts; and the safe use of medical devices (Healthcare Commission, 2009). The investigation identified ineffective reporting of incidents, with the reported information often of poor quality, making it difficult to learn from incidents. It was also found that trusts did not always review and update policies in the light of safety alerts. The Commission recommended that more attention be paid to the proactive identification of risks to safe care, rather than responding only after incidents have occurred (Healthcare Commission, 2009).

Theoretical aspects of patient safety

Evidence-based practice is important in patient safety. Muir Gray (2004) traced developments in evidence-based healthcare. Against the background of financial pressures in the 1970s the emphasis was on efficiency and *doing things cheaper*. During the 1980s rising public expectations led to an emphasis on quality improvement and *doing things better*. The combination of these two approaches formed the drive *to do things right*, supported, for example, by clinical audit. In the twenty-first century, with the focus on available evidence, the emphasis is on *doing the right things right*, informed by the need to *do more good than harm* (Muir Gray, 2004).

But as well as using evidence, the delivery of healthcare relies on a series of complex interactions between people. With increasing complexity in healthcare delivery, the potential for errors and consequent harm expands. Errors are costly for patients and healthcare professionals (Kohn et al., 2000). Patients lose trust in the system, experience longer periods in hospital with physical and psychological discomfort; healthcare professionals experience dissatisfaction and frustration at not being able to provide the best possible care (Kohn et al., 2000).

Errors occur as either *errors of execution*, when the correct action is chosen but it does not proceed as intended, or as *errors of planning*, when the chosen action is not the correct one (Reason, 1990). Designing safe systems requires understanding of the sources of errors and how to design systems to prevent or minimise these errors (Kohn et al., 2000).

Activity 5.2   *Critical thinking*

Can you think of examples of errors of execution and errors of planning?

There is a brief outline answer at the end of the chapter.

Even when the correct procedure for administration of medicines is known and followed, errors of execution can occur if distractions prevent the procedure from continuing as intended. Errors of planning can arise if practice is not based on evidence, or if an incorrect decision is made about patient care – for example, a nurse takes an elderly patient to the toilet, leaves them unattended, and the patient falls from the toilet and suffers a bone fracture. These are human errors.

Concept summary: human error

Reason (1990, p9) defines error as *a generic term to encompass all those occasions in which a planned sequence of mental or physical activities fails to achieve its intended outcome, and when these failures cannot be attributed to the intervention of some chance agency.* Reason identifies two types of errors.

- Active errors are those that are immediately apparent.
- Latent errors arise from adverse consequences that lie dormant within a system for a long time.

Through analysing in detail major accidents such as Bhopal and Chernobyl, Reason suggests that latent errors pose the greatest threat to the safety of complex systems. Reason uses the metaphor of *resident pathogen* (p197) to illustrate this notion of risk factors that are present in any system. Existing latent errors allow active errors to occur when combined with other factors. The more complex a system is, the more resident pathogens are likely to exist.

Reason's work has led to an emphasis on a 'safety culture' that encourages people to openly report safety incidents so that they can be analysed and similar problems avoided in the future. This safety culture replaces a 'culture of blame', which can encourage people to cover up safety incidents for fear of retribution. A blame culture does not help in putting unsafe acts in context, so lessons are not learned for the future. However, even if we focus on how an unsafe act occurred, this does not absolve individuals from being called to account for poor practice.

Application of theory and policy to practice

You will now examine some stories of people with learning disabilities who received inadequate care and treatment from hospitals and social care services (MENCAP, 2007).

Case study: *Death by indifference* (MENCAP, 2007)

The report by MENCAP Death by indifference *presents stories of six people with learning disabilities who died while receiving health and social care services. MENCAP believes that these people died unnecessarily, as a result of institutional discrimination. The stories include the following.*

Martin had a severe learning disability and died in hospital at the age of 43. Martin was admitted to hospital following a stroke; he could not speak or swallow. Speech and language therapists advised that he should not attempt to eat or drink anything, and alternative feeding methods should be established. Martin did receive intravenous fluids, but he sometimes pulled out the cannula. No other attempts were made to provide Martin with nutrition. By the time a decision was made to insert a gastrostomy tube to feed Martin (21 days after admission to hospital), he was too weak to undergo an operation. He died five days later.

Tom died in hospital at the age of 20. Tom had profound and multiple learning disabilities; he began to show signs of distress while at a residential special school. Tom's parents insisted that he receive medical investigations, as they believed he was in pain. A consultant suggested that the pain was related to Tom's digestive system and recommended investigations; however, these did not take place. Following school, Tom was placed in an NHS psychiatric unit, then an adult care home. Tom's health continued to deteriorate; he lost weight and exhibited unusual behaviour. He was eventually admitted to hospital, where an ulcerated oesophagus was diagnosed. An operation was performed to insert a gastrostomy feeding tube, but Tom died before feeding commenced as he was extremely weak.

These are summaries of two of the six stories contained in MENCAP's report. The full stories can be found in the report on MENCAP's website, www.mencap.org.uk, and also in the report by the Ombudsman (Parliamentary and Health Service Ombudsman, 2009). Martin's story was also reported in national newspapers (for example, Carvel, 2009). MENCAP asked the Parliamentary and Health Service Ombudsman to investigate complaints about the care received by the six patients, on behalf of their families. This is an independent service that investigates complaints against government departments and public agencies in the UK and the NHS in England. The Ombudsman's report can be found on the website: www.ombudsman.org.uk/improving-public-service/reports-and-consultations. Investigations by the Ombudsman into the deaths of these six people with learning disabilities identified significant failures across health and social care services. The Ombudsman upheld the complaint that the person concerned was treated less favourably in some aspects of their care and treatment in four out of the six cases (Parliamentary and Health Service Ombudsman, 2009).

Activity 5.3   *Team working*

Read the summaries of the above two stories again. Can you see any common factors in these two stories that might have contributed to the patients' safety being compromised?

What areas of policy are relevant in these stories?

There is a brief outline answer at the end of the chapter.

The Ombudsman investigated each complaint individually but identified some common areas of concern. These included: communication; partnership working and coordination; relationships with families and carers; failure to follow routine procedures; quality of management; and advocacy. You will have identified at least some of these yourself in your answer to the activity. There is no shortage of policy and good practice guidance relating to the health and social care of people with learning disabilities. We will now consider some of these policies.

Policies relating to feeding patients

It is clear from the two brief summaries that both patients were malnourished. NICE provides guidance for nutritional support in adults (NICE, 2006b). The guidance states that screening for risk of malnutrition should take place on admission for hospital patients, at the first clinic appointment for outpatients, and on admission to care homes. Patients are considered at risk of malnutrition if they have eaten little or nothing for more than five days. A screening tool such as the Malnutrition Universal Screening Tool (MUST) should be used, and if patients are considered to be at risk of malnutrition, oral, enteral or parenteral nutritional support should be considered. The guidance states that all acute trusts should have a multidisciplinary nutrition support team, which should include a specialist nutrition support nurse. As well as supporting nursing colleagues, the role of the nurse also extends to community support.

Policies relating to people with learning disabilities

An increasing number of people with learning disabilities live into adulthood and old age and, as a consequence of co-morbidities, are high and frequent users of health services (Brown et al., 2010; Phillips, 2012). Policies for people with learning disabilities reflect a rights-based approach and promote the use of mainstream services wherever possible, while not negating the need for specialist services. General health and social care services therefore face increasing demand for their services by people with learning disabilities. However, evidence suggests that there is indifference to meeting the needs of this group of people in general healthcare services (MENCAP, 2007; Brown et al., 2010; Phillips, 2012).

There has been a move away from institutional care for people with learning disabilities towards policy that promotes and enables more inclusive and ordinary lives (Brown et al., 2010). Brown et al. state that each of the four countries of the UK has produced policies that aim to support this trend:

- *The same as you?* (Scottish Executive, 2000)
- *Fulfilling the promises* (Learning Disability Advisory Group, 2001)
- *Equal lives* (DHSSPS, 2005)
- *Valuing people now* (DH, 2009b)
  (Brown et al., 2010, p353)

The DH (2009b) acknowledges that people with learning disabilities have poorer health than the rest of the population and shorter life expectancies. Their access to the NHS is often poor and characterised by problems that undermine *personalisation, dignity and safety*. The strategy *Valuing people now* (DH, 2009b) conveys a commitment to the human rights of people with learning disabilities and calls on the NHS to reduce inequalities through the improvement of services for people with learning disabilities.

The Ombudsman's report on the care and treatment of the six patients with learning disabilities found evidence in some cases of NHS trusts not making reasonable adjustments to the organisation and delivery of care in order to accommodate the special needs of these individuals (Parliamentary and Health Service Ombudsman, 2009).

In response to the policy imperative to improve the care and treatment of people with learning disabilities in hospitals, Gaskell and Nightingale (2010) describe how, through partnership working between health facilitators and a hospital trust, access to health services by people with learning disabilities was improved. Health facilitators visited people with learning disabilities to ensure access to health services when needed. Patient-held health records were created, which served as communication tools when accessing health services, including acute care. Educational events were held for trust staff on awareness of learning disabilities. Resource folders were provided to wards, containing information on management of patients with learning disabilities, details for assistance, care pathways, flow charts and communication tools.

Policy relating to interprofessional and partnership working

We have already considered interprofessional working in Chapters 2 and 3, and it is clear from the two summaries of the stories that there was poor communication between members of the multidisciplinary teams in health and social services. But there was also a lack of partnership working with the families and carers of the patients. The Ombudsman report explains how people with a learning disability can find it difficult to communicate their symptoms and to understand what is being said to them. In such cases the role of the usual carers in interpreting changes in behaviour is crucial. The lack of collaborative working without doubt contributed to a failure to detect deterioration in the patients.

In the case of Martin, the Ombudsman service found that the hospital trust had not followed national and professional recommendations regarding the care of people who have suffered strokes. The *National stroke strategy* (DH, 2007) states that every local area should provide specialist stroke services, and NICE guidelines for stroke (NICE, 2008) state that people who have experienced an acute stroke and are unable to take adequate nutrition and fluids orally should receive feeding with a naso-gastric tube within 24 hours of admission.

Activity 5.4   *Leadership and management*

Now that you have considered the omissions in the care of these two patients, can you think of any latent errors that contributed to the occurrence of active errors?

There is a brief outline answer at the end of the chapter.

It is likely that the latent conditions of lack of awareness of policy and legislation concerning the care of people with learning disabilities, together with poor interprofessional communication, contributed to the active errors of failing to recognise, and act on, deterioration in these patients. We will now explore failures in communication as contributory factors to patient safety incidents.

Failings in communication and multidisciplinary team working

Failure in communication is a frequent cause of patient safety incidents (Beaumont et al., 2008). We have already seen how effective communication and teamwork is essential for the delivery of high-quality, safe patient care (Leonard et al., 2004). Evidence exists of the barriers to effective interprofessional working within multi-professional healthcare teams. These barriers include professional culture, professional identity, professional status, language and value systems (Hudson, 2002; Johnson et al., 2003; Baxter and Brumfitt, 2008). These barriers can also be exacerbated by a lack of shared language and values within multicultural healthcare teams. Pahor and Rasmussen (2009) identify cultural differences between Swedish and Slovenian healthcare professionals regarding teamwork and relationships between professions, as well as in respect of the 'right thing' to do in relation to patients' problems.

> **Research summary: How does culture show? A case study of an international and interprofessional course in palliative care**
>
> Pahor and Rasmussen (2009) describe a study that aimed to develop innovative forms of palliative care education through an international, interprofessional and IT-supported undergraduate course for Swedish and Slovenian students of nursing, medicine, occupational therapy, physiotherapy, psychology and social work. The course specifically aimed to address differences in professional and national cultures relevant to quality in palliative care. The researchers acknowledge that there are different professional cultures, as well as different national cultures but also recognise that there are different cultural beliefs attached to death and dying. With increasing numbers of deaths occurring in hospitals or other institutions, it is important that healthcare professionals understand cultural differences. Qualitative analysis of evaluation materials from students, teachers and an external evaluation study found that students were able to learn about other professions as a consequence of the interprofessional nature of the course. Cultural differences were not very pronounced between Swedish and Slovenian participants, except in relation to teamwork and relationships between professionals (Slovenian society is generally more hierarchical than Swedish society) and in relation to the 'right thing' to do in relation to patients' problems. The example of what to do for a patient who would not eat arose in the research; there were differences in what was considered appropriate practice in such a case, with the practice of force feeding being more familiar in Slovenia than in Sweden.

Similarly, many non-UK qualified doctors find that the ethical framework within which healthcare is practised in the UK is different from that of their country of qualification (Slowther et al., 2009). Commenting on the globalisation of healthcare, Fortier (2008) claims that growing diversity *has deep implications for how care is designed, delivered and received* (p87) and affects those who deliver care as well as those on the receiving end. Health professionals have been found to experience uncertainty and apprehension in responding to the needs of patients of cultures that are different from their own (Kai et al., 2007). Patients from minority cultures and those who do not speak the language of the host country are disproportionately at risk of experiencing preventable adverse events while in hospital compared to the host population (Johnstone and Kanitsaki, 2006). Johnstone and Kanitsaki argue that there is a need to recognise the critical relationship between culture, language and safety, and quality of care. Fortier (2008, p87) refers to a meeting convened by the International Centre for Migration and Health, where people from different countries differed with respect to *terminology, conceptual frameworks, organisational constraints and political realities.*

According to Cambridge (2008, p166), three components of safety are: a safe product; safe systems (governance); and a safe professional workforce (professional regulation). While the benefits of a diverse workforce are recognised (NMC, 2011), several challenges are posed by multicultural healthcare teams (Alexis, 2005; Hearnden, 2008) – for example, communication, the need to maintain cohesion in the presence of cultural differences and the individual needs of the team members. Smith et al. (2006) report that overseas-trained nurses are over-represented in cases of clinical malpractice reported to the NMC, arguing that this is related to insufficient diversity awareness and a lack of recognition of non-British healthcare experience and expertise. Cowan and Norman (2006) argue that courses designed to enhance cultural competence form a vital part of induction programmes for migrant nurses in order to facilitate their integration into multicultural healthcare teams, while Gijón-Sánchez et al. (2010) recommend intercultural competence training for all health professionals in the EU.

Improving interprofessional communication

One important opportunity for multidisciplinary teams to engage in detailed discussions concerning their patients is the ward round. This has sometimes been neglected amid pressures to fulfil heavy workloads. It is during ward rounds that doctors make decisions about the care and treatment of their patients, and a full understanding of a patient's progress can only be reached if other members of the multidisciplinary team are present and contributing to the discussion. So important is the ward round to safe, effective and high-quality patient care that the Royal College of Physicians and the Royal College of Nursing joined forces to produce guidance for best practice for ward rounds (RCP and RCN, 2012). The guidance states that ward rounds need to be prioritised and that the presence of a senior nurse is essential; nurses have a key role to play in ward rounds in terms of sharing information, supporting patients and ensuring continuity of care. The guidance can be reviewed at www.rcplondon.ac.uk; search for 'Ward rounds in medicine: principles for best practice', and then engage in the following activity.

Activity 5.5   *Decision-making*

Arrange to attend a multidisciplinary ward round in your placement. How do the various professionals on the round communicate? What sort of information do they contribute to discussions about the patients' care? What types of decisions are made about patients' care? Are the patients involved in the decision-making? How does the ward round contribute to patient safety?

There is a brief outline answer at the end of the chapter.

The guidance indicates that ward rounds should include a holistic assessment of the patient, with priority being given to the quality and safety of care, and an appreciation of the patient's experience. We will now turn to the recognition of deterioration in patients.

Recognising deterioration in patients

The NPSA is the leading agency on national initiatives to improve patient safety. The NPSA achieves this through the NRLS, which collects reports on incidents from healthcare staff across

England and Wales, and provides a national database for patient safety incidents. These are used to analyse trends and make recommendations for action (Beaumont et al., 2008). Analysis of reported serious incidents resulting in death during 2005 revealed patient deterioration as a key theme (Beaumont et al., 2008). A report *Safer care for the acutely ill patient: learning from serious incidents* (NPSA, 2007) contains analysis of 64 deaths related to failure to detect or act on deterioration in patients; contributory factors included failure to notice changes in patients' conditions as a result of inadequate recording of observations, failure to recognise the importance of deterioration, and delay in securing medical attention when deterioration was detected (Beaumont et al., 2008). There were also failures in communication. Once it was recognised that detecting deterioration in patients can reduce morbidity, mortality and length of hospital stay, there was a series of related policy documents, including NICE guidelines *Acutely ill patients in hospital: recognition of and response to acute illness in adults in hospital* (NICE, 2007). The key to detecting deterioration in patients are observation tools that prompt calculation of early warning scores that in turn indicate appropriate action to be taken.

National Early Warning Score (NEWS)

While there are a number of early warning scores in use across the NHS, the lack of standardisation of these tools means that as staff move around the NHS they have to familiarise themselves with different tools (RCP, 2012a). A consistent approach to the detection of changes in a patient's condition is desirable, and the Royal College of Physicians commissioned a multidisciplinary group to develop a National Early Warning Score (NEWS) for universal use with adults. The score consists of six physiological measurements: respiratory rate, oxygen saturations, temperature, systolic blood pressure, pulse rate and level of consciousness (RCP, 2012a). The full report provides guidance on interpreting the recorded measurements and appropriate clinical responses.

From patient safety to trust

Trust in healthcare can be reduced when expectations are not met. Trust is an essential part of being a professional and entails *letting other persons . . . take care of something that the truster cares about* (Frowe, 2005, pp34–5). In this case health is generally highly valued. Trusting relationships between healthcare professionals are more likely to result in successful outcomes; the message from politicians, the media, professionals and the public is that trust matters (Brownlie and Howson, 2008). Calnan and Rowe (2008) suggest that trust has emerged as a quality indicator and that a trustor expects a trustee to work in their best interests. Yet, trust in healthcare professionals may be called into question against the background of media reports of adverse events in the NHS. In the 1990s, attention was drawn to mortality from **iatrogenic illness** (Entwistle and Quick, 2006); Harold Shipman, the GP who murdered many of his elderly female patients during the period 1974–1988, was eventually confirmed as Britain's worst mass murderer (Leppard, 2002); more recently, there have been reports of failure to meet the needs of elderly patients (Parliamentary and Health Service Ombudsman, 2011). In spite of these reports, research in the UK suggests that, generally speaking, patients have retained their trust in individual clinicians (Calnan and Rowe, 2008). However, there is a growing concern over reduced public trust in healthcare systems, reflecting changes in the organisation of healthcare delivery, particularly when cost-cutting measures are in place (Mechanic and Meyer, 2000; Calnan and Sanford, 2004).

Concept summary: trust

Trust is grounded in relations (Gilson, 2003; Mechanic and Meyer, 2000), and is only required when there is some uncertainty and some degree of risk (Brown, 2008; Calnan and Rowe, 2008). When an individual is placed in a position that requires placing trust in another person, he will assimilate available information and make a decision whether or not to enter into a trusting relationship (Johns, 1996). Möllering (2001, p412) likens this to a mental process of leaping *across the gorge of the unknowable from the land of interpretation into the land of expectation.* The expectation of entering a trusting relationship is that the outcome will be favourable.

We will now explore a case study concerning a group of **refugees** and **asylum seekers** from the Democratic Republic of Congo (DRC) living in London (Taylor, 2007). Refugees and asylum seekers are among the poor and vulnerable groups in society, and the poorer people are, the less able they are to access the information that allows the pursuit of 'informed' trust (Rowe and Calnan, 2006). MORI (2003) confirms that loss of trust is more pronounced among members of black and minority ethnic groups than among the white majority population in the UK.

Case study: Etienne

Etienne has been in London for several years. He is married and has two children; his family are with him in London. Etienne has refugee status in the UK. He is 37 years old. He was a jeweller in the DRC and he lived in the capital city Kinshasa. He does not have employment in the UK, but he is studying languages, so he does speak some English. Etienne generally describes himself as healthy, though he sometimes experiences headaches. He worries about the situation in the DRC, and has concerns for family and friends who are still there. Etienne chose to bring his family to London as he felt it would be safer.

During a social meeting of members of the Congolese community at Etienne's home, there was a discussion concerning their experiences of using healthcare services in London. Etienne was expressing some disappointment with healthcare, telling his friends that every time to goes to his GP the very most common thing they prescribe you is paracetamol. *A friend responded:* Yes, the same thing they will give for any kind of illness; *and then another friend said:* Always paracetamol. *Etienne's wife, Florence, told a story of her young son and how, when he was a baby, a health visitor told her that the boy had problems with hearing, but when the GP examined the boy he said that her son could hear, and that he could find nothing abnormal. However, the family is still receiving letters from the hospital offering an appointment to assess the boy's hearing. Florence said:* It's confusing – who shall we trust? *Another friend, Robert, expressed the fear that refugees and asylum seekers are being experimented on in British hospitals; a female friend was concerned that a series of repeat cervical smears was forming part of an experiment.*

continued . . . •••

When asked if he trusted the healthcare professionals, Etienne replied: When my English was very little I used to try to trust them, but now watching some programmes on TV, and I'm reading some newspaper . . . there are so many doctors killing people, giving them wrong tablets . . . so most of the time I have to be careful.

Activity 5.6	*Critical thinking*

It is clear from the above case study that there is considerable lack of trust among this group of refugees and asylum seekers concerning healthcare providers and services. Why do think this might be?

There is a brief outline answer at the end of the chapter.

Refugees, asylum seekers and trust

There are specific reasons why refugees and asylum seekers might not feel able to trust healthcare providers and services. Lack of trust permeates the entire 'refugee experience' and endures into the post-settlement period (Hynes, 2003). Ager defines the 'refugee experience' as *the human consequences – personal, social, economic, cultural and political – of forced migration* (Ager, 1999, p2).

Experiences in the home country and/or during flight may initiate a protective mechanism in the form of a failure to trust a range of people, including healthcare professionals. It has been known for refugees and asylum seekers to be betrayed by neighbours and acquaintances in their home countries (Ager, 1999), and by teachers, doctors and nurses who have been forced to betray patients or others sheltering in hospitals (Summerfield, 1999).

It is important that nurses do not become defensive if faced with patients who appear to be suspicious of them. Gilson (2003) notes that trust is unequally distributed in societies and that more powerful people are more likely to be trusting; as a consequence of a *less positive world view* (Gilson, 2003, p1459) those who are socially excluded trust less readily. Indeed, according to Muecke (1992), suspicion is a survival skill for refugees and asylum seekers. Suspicion also influences behaviour towards professionals, and it is evident how, for refugees and asylum seekers, lack of trust can be extended to healthcare professionals, who may be viewed as agents of the state and potential collaborators in the immigration process. The lack of trust may also be compounded by difficulty in communicating with healthcare professionals and lack of knowledge about the NHS and how it operates.

Policy, trust and safety

The complexity of modern healthcare systems contributes to patient safety problems (Entwistle and Quick, 2006). In general, policy responses to the problems of safety and public trust include:

learning from past safety incidents; designing technology and healthcare systems to reduce the risks of safety incidents; implementing early warning systems; reporting measures to improve patient safety; greater transparency in the regulation of the healthcare professions; and ensuring safety features in professional education programmes (Entwistle and Quick, 2006).

Such has been the government concern over declining trust in the NHS that a White Paper *Trust, assurance and safety: the regulation of health professionals in the 21st century* (Secretary of State for Health, 2007) sets out a programme of reform for England's system for the regulation of health professionals, requiring – among other things – increasing lay membership on governing bodies, greater accountability of these bodies to Parliament, and measures for ensuring fitness to practise, all within the broader framework of clinical governance.

Regulation and the nursing profession

The Council membership of the NMC consists of seven lay members and seven professional members. The *Code* (NMC, 2008) is a key tool in safeguarding the health and wellbeing of the public and *as such establishes the bar for fitness to practise* (House of Commons Health Committee, 2011). Employers, professionals and members of the public can make a formal referral to the NMC if they think that a nurse or midwife is in breach of the code. Government departments have select committees that are appointed by the House of Commons with the remit of examining the expenditure, administration and policy of the relevant department. The Health Committee raised concerns about the recent dramatic rise in the numbers of referrals of nurses and midwives to the NMC; during the three years 2008–2011 there was a 102-per-cent increase in referrals about nurses and midwives (House of Commons Health Committee, 2011). Further concern was expressed that the NMC does not know why referrals are increasing.

Consequences of failure to comply with policy on safety

The Health Committee expressed concern about the standard of basic nursing care for older people in hospital, and the Health Service Ombudsman raised significant issues with the care of older people, particularly in acute hospitals. In response to declining standards of care, the NMC published guidance to the professions on the care of older people (NMC, 2009). However, the Health Committee was disappointed with the response from nursing and midwifery professions. The committee also noted that, despite the poor standards of care found in some areas of the Mid Staffordshire NHS Foundation Trust, not one nurse or midwife had reported concerns to the NMC (House of Commons Health Committee, 2011). The consequence for professional staff of the Mid Staffordshire Trust is that the NMC has dealt with approximately 40 fitness to practise cases. The Health Committee has urged the NMC to send a clear reminder to nurses and midwives of the consequences of failure to report poor practice. The NMC has also been charged with the development of an action plan to improve the care of older people.

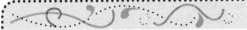

Chapter summary

Patient safety is what social scientists call a 'wicked problem' – that is, one that is *messy, persistent and multidimensional* (Braithwaite et al., 2009). We have seen in this chapter that patient safety is an important and enduring component of the overall quality agenda of health policy. While individual healthcare professionals remain responsible and accountable for their own actions, the general trend is to create a safety culture by learning from mistakes and looking for weaknesses in healthcare systems rather than blaming individuals. We have explored stories of patients with learning disabilities in order to illustrate the tragic consequences of failure to adhere to safety procedures as well as provide compassionate care. We have also considered how concerns about safety can result in a lack of trust in healthcare systems and professionals, particularly in relation to vulnerable people. However, lack of trust is not confined to vulnerable groups.

Activities: Brief outline answers

Activity 5.1: Leadership and management (page 83)

You might have identified the following.

- Local policy on incident reporting.
- A local patient safety champion.
- Training programmes for patient safety.
- Risk assessment procedures.
- Local policy for communication with patients and their families when an incident has occurred.

Activity 5.2: Critical thinking (page 84)

You might have identified an error of execution when the correct procedure is followed for the administration of medicines, but an emergency situation prevents the administration being completed. An error of planning can arise when the choice of action is not based on evidence.

Activity 5.3: Team working (page 86)

Both of the patients were clearly malnourished, so you might have identified failure to follow policies relating to feeding patients. You will probably have identified failure to adhere to policies concerning effective interprofessional working, and working in partnership with families and carers. You might have identified failure to adhere to policies and laws relating to the treatment of people with learning disabilities.

Activity 5.4: Leadership and management (page 88)

Latent errors include lack of awareness about policy and legislation concerning the care of people with learning disabilities, together with apparent weak interprofessional communication. It is likely that both of these conditions contributed to the active error of failing to feed the patients.

Activity 5.5: Decision-making (page 90)

You will have identified that contributions from the various professionals relate to the progress that the patient is making, and allow the consultant to assess the effectiveness, or otherwise, of the treatment plan.

Patient safety should be enhanced by ensuring that care and treatment is going to plan and there are no gaps, or misunderstandings, in the patient's overall care plan. Decisions made at ward rounds often have to be conveyed to other professionals or family members. Attendance at, and involvement in, the ward round can ensure that the correct information is passed on to other care providers.

Activity 5.6: Critical thinking (page 93)

You may have noted that there may be misunderstandings as a consequence of lack of familiarity with the NHS in the UK. There may have been problems with communication with healthcare providers; while the refugees and asylum seekers spoke some English, they may not always have been able to communicate meaningfully with healthcare providers. You will also have noted that Etienne was aware of media reports of adverse events in the NHS.

You may be aware that there are also specific reasons why refugees and asylum seekers may not feel able to trust healthcare providers – these are discussed in the chapter.

Further reading

Beaumont, K, Luettel, D and Thomson, R (2008) Deterioration in hospital patients: early signs and appropriate actions. *Nursing Standard*, 23(1): 43–8.

This article describes the role of the NPSA and discusses some patient safety incidents identified by analysis of reports of serious incidents.

Brown, M, MacArthur, J, McKechanie, A, Hayes, M and Fletcher, J (2010) Equality and access to general health care for people with learning disabilities: reality or rhetoric? *Journal of Research in Nursing*, 15(4): 351–61.

This article provides an interesting analysis of policy relating to people with learning disabilities.

MENCAP (2012) *Out of sight: stopping the neglect and abuse of people with a learning disability*. Available at: **www.mencap.org.uk/outofsight.**

This report describes the neglect of people with learning disabilities in institutions.

Phillips, L (2012) Improving care for people with learning disabilities in hospital. *Nursing Standard*, 26(23): 42–8.

This article provides a literature review identifying inequalities in relation to the care and treatment of people with learning disabilities in hospital and making recommendations for improvement.

Useful website

www.npsa.nhs.uk

The National Patient Safety Agency website provides reports on safety incidents and guidance to promote patient safety.

Chapter 6
The policy context of care, compassion and dignity

Chapter aims

After reading this chapter, you will be able to:

*   discuss the social construction of caring within health policy;
*   recognise the importance of the contribution of informal carers to society;
*   critically analyse how theoretical aspects of caring can be related to nursing practice;
*   draw on, and learn from, reports of failings in care in order contribute to the continuous drive to improve the quality of care through nursing practice;
*   recognise the part that nurses can play in contributing to policy that aims to improve the quality of care.

Introduction

Scenario: Ellen

Ellen Franks is 64 years old. Two years ago she was diagnosed with lung cancer and following treatment was able to return to her normal way of life. Recently she has been experiencing pain in her chest. Initially, she did not do anything about it, hoping it would go away; she was worried about the cancer returning and frightened of going into hospital again. She has now accepted that something is wrong and has been admitted to an assessment ward. Ellen was very anxious on admission, but has now told her relatives: The nurse who attended to me was caring and thoughtful. She immediately gave me some medication that the doctor had prescribed and that has relieved the pain – I have confidence in the staff now. I feel more at ease.

This is an example of good practice; a caring nurse has been able to allay this patient's anxiety and gain her confidence. Sadly, this is not always the case, and in this chapter we will look at some of the reports of failings in care that have forced caring on to the healthcare policy agenda. We will also consider how the nursing profession is responding and contributing to policy development in relation to caring.

This chapter will address policy related to caring. We will start by looking at the wider policy context of caring by considering informal carers, identifying how the notion of 'carer' is socially constructed and how it has increasingly become important in policy. The chapter will then address some theoretical aspects of caring, and this will lead into a discussion concerning caring and the nursing profession. We will look at political interventions in what might be deemed nursing policy, particularly surrounding compassion and dignity. We will revisit Ivy's case study to illustrate how policy and guidelines relating to dignity can be applied in practice.

We will start by thinking about theoretical aspects of care and caring.

Defining care

Care is an activity that is central to nursing, but it is not unique to nursing – there are other caring professions. During your nursing education you will no doubt have come across several definitions of 'care' and also engaged in discussions surrounding the nature of care. This chapter concerns policy relating to care and will start with the wider context of care, which has attracted policy attention for some time, before addressing policy relating to nursing care, which has not featured prominently in the policy agenda until recently.

The following definition of care comes from policy literature – indeed, from an article titled 'Care as a good for social policy':

Care . . . refers to looking after those who cannot take care of themselves. It can be defined as the activities and relations involved in caring for the ill, elderly and dependent young.
(Daly, 2002, p252)

In her article, Mary Daly considers the relationship between policy, care and society, describing how characteristic features of care may include notions of moral orientation and of labour. It is hardly surprising that care has become a key concern of social policy (Fink, 2004). When the welfare state was established in the 1940s, it was formed with the assumption of a 'male breadwinner' model, which entailed a male head of household who went out to work to earn money in order to support his family, and a wife who stayed at home and cared for her husband, children and the general household. Care was very much the province of women and was to a great extent taken for granted. This traditional reliance on women as providers of care led to care becoming *one of the original feminist concepts* (Daly, 2002, p252) as feminist writers drew attention to the consequences of unpaid domestic labour for women. While such writings raised the issue of women's situation within the informal and private setting of the family, the role of the state in relation to deriving benefit from this tradition was not overlooked. Over time, changing demographic, economic and cultural factors in the form of an ageing population, together with the increasing number of women in paid work and diverse family structures, have brought care into the policy arena as the male breadwinner model ceased to be dominant. These changes have resulted in increasing numbers of people needing support from the state in order to meet their needs for care.

Informal carers

Activity 6.1   *Reflection*

Think about your current or recent clinical placement. Who were the 'carers' of your patients when they were at home? Who provided information about your patient? Who did the nurses communicate with about discharge plans?

There is a brief outline answer at the end of the chapter.

This activity leads us into the realm of informal carers. The nature of your chosen placement might have led you to identify different types of carers, depending on whether the placement was for adults, children, acutely ill people, those with long-term conditions or those with mental health problems. Nevertheless, these carers might have some features in common. It is likely that the majority of carers are women, though there are a substantial number of men carers, and also young people and even children. The following information about informal carers has been collected by Carers UK, an organisation that aims to improve the lives of carers and – through campaigns and the provision of information – raise the profile of the contribution that carers make to society.

Facts about carers

The following facts are drawn from a report called *Facts about carers*, and the figures provided come from the 2001 Census (Carers UK, 2009).

- There are nearly 6 million carers in the UK, representing 10 per cent of the total population.

- In the UK there are 3,400,000 female carers (58 per cent of carers) and 2,460,000 male carers (42 per cent of carers).
- Women are more likely to relinquish paid work in order to care.
- Most carers are over the age of 18.
- More than 1 in 5 people are found in the peak age range for caring, which is 50–59 years.
- 174,995 young people under the age of 18 years of age are providing care; 85 per cent of these provide care for 1–19 hours per week. However, 13,029 of these young people engage in caring activities for 50 hours or more per week.
- Concerning minority ethnic groups, Bangladeshi and Pakistani men and women are three times more likely to provide care compared with white British men and women.

It is clear that a lot of people are caring for dependent family members, providing a vital resource for society. It has been estimated that the value of the contribution made by carers amounts to £119 billion per year (Carers UK, 2011). It is not surprising, then, that governments have been keen to harness this support, and that as women's roles and family structures have changed, the whole business of providing care has received increasing policy attention. While assessing and meeting the needs of carers is the remit of local authorities, nurses need to take into account carers' situations when planning for discharging patients to their homes. It is also important not to make assumptions about carers. The following activity invites you to consider the implications of caring.

Activity 6.2   *Critical thinking*

What might the consequences be for people who engage in caring activities over long periods of time?

What are the implications of women giving up work to care?

There is a brief outline answer at the end of the chapter.

There can be consequences for the mental and physical health of anyone who provides care for a dependent family member, or friend, over long periods of time if they do not have adequate support. Women who give up work are at risk of experiencing loss of earnings and loss of, or reduction in, an occupational pension. This can have serious consequences in later life. We will consider a case study of a woman who struggled single-handedly to care for her dependent mother.

Case study: Sarah Mills

Sarah Mills is a 52-year-old head teacher at a primary school. She lives with her elderly mother, who is 84 years old and has very restricted mobility due to arthritis. Sarah adores her mother and has promised her that she will never let her be placed in residential care. She sees it as both a duty and an honour to care for her mother. But Sarah also has a successful career, and she has worked hard to achieve and maintain this. The job

---

continued . . .

demands that she works long hours. Sarah is also aware that she needs her career in order to be able to provide for herself in old age. Consequently, she is finding it very difficult to meet the demands of her job and also provide the care needed by her increasingly dependent mother. Sarah is very proud and has not wanted to ask for help; she is also wary of strangers coming into her home to help with her mother's care. Sarah feels that she knows her mother so well that she is best placed to meet her needs.

Nevertheless, Sarah finally reached the stage where she was experiencing extreme stress trying to juggle the demands of the two roles. Colleagues and friends noticed changes in Sarah and became worried for her welfare, and for that of her mother. The colleagues and friends managed to persuade Sarah to contact social services and request an assessment of needs, but before help was forthcoming, Sarah had to stop work because of acute anxiety attacks. At that stage Sarah's mother had to be placed in residential care.

The case study illustrates quite an extreme case of what can happen when carers remain unsupported. We have already seen how Ivy was placed on a waiting list when her daughter requested help from social services, so even when there is a fairly clear case of need for advice, if not support, help is not always immediately available. The case study illustrates that nurses should not make assumptions about the ability of family members to provide care and that nurses should have sufficient policy awareness to be able to make suggestions about appropriate referrals if they suspect that a carer is under pressure. Nurses also have responsibilities in relation to policy concerning safeguarding adults, so they need to know the procedures to be followed if they suspect an adult may be at risk.

Policy and caring

It is estimated that the number of people needing care will soon exceed the number of people who are available and willing to provide care (Carers UK, 2011). Governments thus have a vested interest in making the work of informal carers easier and have acknowledged that carers need support; policy has been put in place to achieve this. However, many people would argue that much more needs to be done to help carers.

Harris (2002) describes how the notion of 'caring' is socially constructed by prevailing political ideologies and resulting policy agendas. Three fairly distinct periods of different health policy agendas can be identified.

First, Harris describes the social democratic approach to the welfare state, which was captured in the work of TH Marshall, which we have already considered in Chapter 4. The nature of the welfare state, as it was established in the 1940s, fostered equality of status, through the provision of universal access to healthcare and enhanced social security arrangements that aimed to provide a subsistence level of income for everyone. Arguably, these rights of social citizenship encouraged a sense of belonging and social solidarity among citizens, and collective obligations for the welfare of other citizens. As we have already seen, this social democratic approach was underpinned by the assumption that men would be the breadwinners while women stayed at home and carried out caring functions. Caring thus formed part of women's unpaid work in the private sphere, viewed as a *taken-for-granted resource* (Harris, 2002, p269) within the informal space of the household.

The next distinctive period of health policy occurred during the 1980s/1990s when the New Right's scepticism towards public services contributed towards measures to reduce expectations of the role of the state in providing for citizens. During this period there was an emphasis on *personal and private, rather than state* responsibilities to provide care (Harris, 2002, p270). Community care policy assumed that most support for people in need of care was provided by family and friends, and such private arrangements became formalised in community care plans and was managed by social workers. This led Harris to claim that care and support within the family moved from being an implicit resource, as perceived within the social democratic model, to an explicit resource under the New Right.

New Labour maintained the reliance on the contribution of informal carers to community care packages. Caring was promoted as an expression of citizenship obligation – or what Daly described as a moral orientation towards caring and a form of **social capital** – within the context of New Labour discourse about the meaning of citizenship and its responsibilities, as caring extends beyond family to society (Sevenhuijsen, 2000; Fink, 2004).

Caring for carers

As caring featured more prominently in policy, its status was raised, and one consequence was the publication of a national carers' strategy (DH, 1999), which promised more support for carers. The Coalition government issued a White Paper on the future of adult social care in 2012. *Caring for our future: reforming care and support* sets out the plans to reform the way people are cared for and supported (Her Majesty's Government, 2012a). Again, the document recognises the needs of an ageing population and acknowledges that everyone will become involved in caring and supporting activities at some time in their life. The White Paper calls for a different approach to caring, arguing that it is not possible to make improvements simply by providing more money for a fragmented care system. Instead, the document states that *society is not making the most of the skills and talents that communities have to offer* (Her Majesty's Government, 2012a, p7). This strongly suggests a continuation of the policy of making the most of informal carers. Indeed, the White Paper refers to mobilising community support in *active communities* where people share their time and skills in order to support fellow community members to maintain independence and wellbeing. The document does acknowledge that improved support for carers is necessary in order to achieve this.

The benefits of caring

Caring should not always be perceived in a bad light – people can gain enormous pleasure and fulfilment from caring for their relatives, and many do see it as a duty. Consider the following case study and research summary. The case study illustrates how carers can be supported in their homes in caring for a dependent relative. The summary draws on research that illustrates the 'feel good' factor that can result from providing support to family members in another country.

Case study: Charlie

Charlie Barnes is in his late 70s and cares for his wife who suffered a stroke and now has limited mobility. Rosie Barnes spends most of her time in a wheelchair – she needs a full-time carer. Charlie takes great pride in caring for his wife, and his role as main carer is made easier by a good support package. As the main carer, Charlie had his own needs assessed when social services assessed his wife's needs for care. Mr and Mrs Barnes receive an attendance allowance, and a personal budget gives them some choice over the services they feel are needed to help them remain in their own home. Adaptations were made to their home to make it suitable for a wheelchair user, carers help with bathing Rosie, and the couple receive some assistance with household tasks. Most importantly, Charlie has been able to employ someone he trusts to sit with Rosie for a few hours a week while he goes out to his local club to enjoy some company with friends and get some respite.

Research summary: 'It is my turn to give': migrants' perceptions of gift exchange and the maintenance of transnational identity

Jane Wangaruro's research focused on Kenyan migrants in the UK and the support – financial and otherwise – that they provide to chronically ill relatives in Kenya. Most African cultures embrace a philosophy that emphasises mutual care within and beyond the family. Consequently, Kenyan migrants in the UK work hard, sometimes with more than one job, to be able to send money and other forms of support home to their relatives in Kenya. Semi-structured interviews were conducted with Kenyan migrants in the UK who were supporting family members remaining in Kenya. As well as investing time in maintaining meaningful relationships with family members, participants talked about the provision of *financial, emotional and spiritual* support. Participants described feeling *satisfied, fulfilled, content* and *just good generally* when they were able to support their ill relatives. Although being able to travel to Kenya to visit their relatives was paramount, the demonstration of caring through sending money and other resources, and through speaking on the phone, provided an intrinsic reward that one participant described as *a good hormone that will make my body healthy . . . their comfort makes me comfortable.* Any sense of obligation to support relatives was balanced by a sense of fulfilment and pride. These acts of caring also helped to maintain identity.

(Taylor et al., 2012)

Although the activities in the above research do not necessarily entail day-to-day caring in the sense described in the previous case study, the research does serve to illustrate that caring acts can be beneficial for the giver as well as the recipient of care. It is also important to be aware that as we live and work in an increasingly multicultural environment, acts such as supporting family members in countries overseas are important to migrants in the UK, be they fellow healthcare professionals or patients, and policy that interferes with their ability to do so may result in distress.

Theorising caring

We have considered the wider policy agenda that addresses caring roles in society. Now we turn our attention to some of the more theoretical aspects of caring. Again, this section will feature literature from the wider policy field, as well as from the discipline of nursing. Ungerson (1987) distinguished between caring *about* and caring *for*, claiming that the person who engages in a caring role may or may not have any emotional commitment to the person they are caring for. Put simply, people who 'do' caring may not 'feel' caring. This is an area that has become important for the nursing profession in the light of widely publicised incidents of failings in caring duties. NHS London (2012) took the decision to reduce the numbers of places available for nurse training in London in the light of meeting the needs of a qualified nurse workforce in London in the next few years, but also with the express intention of training fewer nurses, but to a higher standard. This came about as a result of senior nurses in London hospital trusts claiming that some students had poor numeracy and literacy skills, and also had poor attitudes towards patients. It was felt that more stringent entry requirements and better educational preparation are needed in order to improve the quality of care (NHS London, 2012). Further, amid concern that the 'public service ethic' may have been lost in the nursing profession, Maben and Griffiths (2008) have called for a reconsideration of the role of the nurse in serving the public, and meeting the needs and expectations of patients and their families.

Caring and compassion and dignity

Sadly, worrying reports by Age Concern (2006, 2010) and the Patients Association (2011) have revealed poor care provision to some older patients in hospitals. The Patients Association's helpline team hears reports of poor care of elderly patients on an almost daily basis, mostly relating to fundamental aspects of care such as communication, toileting, pain relief, nutrition and hydration, providing examples of systematic failings in the NHS (Patients Association, 2011). Against the background of such reports, the Secretary of State for Health asked the CQC to look at standards of dignity in hospitals. The reports of the CQC's inspections revealed cases of hospitals in England that were failing to meet their legal obligations to provide basic standards in relation to dignity and nutrition for older patients. In one case a clinician had to prescribe water to a patient to ensure that they received adequate hydration (Campbell, 2011).

The Care Quality Commission's inspections

The CQC made 100 unannounced inspections of acute NHS hospitals in England. The inspection teams included practising nurses and people with experience of care services. During the inspections the teams observed the delivery of care on the hospital wards, talked to patients and their families and interviewed staff. The inspection teams focused on standards of dignity and nutrition on wards caring for elderly people (CQC, 2011a).

The CQC's report (2011a) acknowledges many examples of good practice and of commitment to patient-centred care. However, the report reveals that concerns were raised in around half of the hospitals inspected, and 20 hospitals were failing to provide care to the standards required by law. The care provided at two hospitals placed people at *unacceptable risk of harm* (CQC, 2011a, p4).

Three key themes in the CQC's findings

The CQC's report's findings revealed three key themes underlying the failings in care.

- There is a need for the creation of a culture in which good care can flourish; this is an element of clinical governance.
- Some staff demonstrated unfortunate attitudes to people – for example, showing lack of respect and not promoting dignity.
- Lack of resources contributed to poor care, but the report stresses that having high staffing levels does not guarantee good care.
(CQC, 2011a)

The findings identify areas that are amenable to improvement through good leadership and management. However, the report also calls upon educators, particularly in nursing, to focus on patient-centred care. Further, the report urges managers to use their budgets wisely in order to support front-line care staff, but the findings also indicate that factors over and above resources are central to the provision of high-quality care, as the inspection teams observed unacceptable care on wards that were well staffed and excellent care on understaffed wards (CQC, 2011a). These findings suggest that there is scope for nurses to take control of professional practice and – through leadership, drive and enthusiasm – to raise standards of care to those seen in the best examples. Examples can be found in the *Time to care* initiative (RCN, 2011b).

Time to care

The RCN's UK-wide Frontline First campaign sought examples of nursing innovation. RCN Wales established a Research and Innovation Unit that seeks to identify innovative examples of good nursing practice and standards of care. For example:

- the Anglesey ward in Morrison Hospital reduced the annual incident rate of pressure ulcers from 4 per cent to zero;
- the Cwm Taf local Health Board introduced a Dignity Pledge for patients, which included displaying 'care in progress' signs when personal procedures are being carried out, ensuring all patients can reach functioning call bells and protecting patient mealtimes.

The Health Service Ombudsman

A report from the Health Service Ombudsman for England (Parliamentary and Health Service Ombudsman, 2011) describes ten investigations into complaints about the standard of care provided to older people by the NHS. The complaints concerned NHS Trusts in England and two GP practices. The Ombudsman reported *a picture of NHS provision that is failing to respond to the needs of older people with care and compassion* (Parliamentary and Health Service Ombudsman, 2011, p8). Worryingly, the report highlighted *a disregard for process and procedure* (p8), which implies a failure to engage with policies. It is instructive to read the report to become familiar with the standards against which the Ombudsman judged the experiences that led to complaints (see 'Useful websites' at the end of the chapter).

Investigations into complaints by the Health Service Ombudsman

A complaint can be referred to the Ombudsman's Office once local attempts to resolve it have been exhausted. The Ombudsman will investigate what should have happened in a particular case and what did actually happen. As well as the Ombudsman's own principles, the standards set out in the NHS Constitution and the principles of human rights – fairness, respect, equality, dignity and autonomy – are used to guide the investigation (Parliamentary and Health Service Ombudsman, 2011).

The NHS Constitution sets out values that should guide the behaviours of those who work in the NHS (DH, 2012b, p14).

- Respect and dignity.
- Commitment to quality of care.
- Compassion.
- Improving lives.
- Working together for patients.
- Everyone counts.

Scenario: Joyce

Joyce is a registered nurse working in a care home for older people. She sometimes feels isolated as there are not many qualified nurses working in the care home, but she enjoys her work as a team leader for a team of health-care assistants. Joyce keeps up to date with policy developments and fulfils her professional responsibility in relation to continuing professional development. She is very concerned about the reports of poor care for older people in hospitals and particularly in care homes. Although she does not work in the NHS – the care home is not part of the NHS – Joyce feels that the values of the NHS Constitution should apply wherever care is practised. She is wondering how she can discuss these values with her team of health care assistants. Joyce has recently read the report from the Commission on Dignity, Delivering dignity: securing dignity in care for older people in hospitals and care homes *(Commission on Dignity in Care, 2012). This document states that team leaders in hospitals and care homes must allow time for staff to reflect on the care they provide and how they can improve. Joyce decides to make time once a week for a team meeting in which her team are encouraged to talk about the care they provide, using the framework of the values of the NHS Constitution. This activity allows Joyce to identify areas where staff development is needed.*

The CQC and Ombudsman Service are powerful organisations, and their reports have been influential in framing policy responses. However, the CQC itself is not beyond reproach and came in for criticism following poor handling of reports of abuse of patients at the former Winterbourne View Hospital, a facility for people with learning disabilities and complex needs (CQC, 2011b). A member of staff reported unacceptable practices to the management of the hospital, South Gloucestershire Adult Safeguarding Team and the CQC, but the response of the CQC and its predecessor, the Healthcare Commission, was inadequate, as judged by the CQC's own internal review (CQC, 2011b). It was left to the BBC *Panorama* programme to expose physical and verbal abuse of patients on national television.

Caring and nursing

Nurses work in complex environments and are expected to provide high-quality care with compassion (Maben and Griffiths, 2008).

Activity 6.3   *Reflection*

At some stage during your educational preparation to become a nurse you will have worked with a qualified nurse who you admired and respected enormously. You will probably have said to yourself, *That is the sort of nurse I want to become.*

Think about one of those expert nurses you have worked with. What was it about that nurse that inspired you to model your professional development on their practice?

There is a brief outline answer at the end of the chapter.

The chances are that you identified a range of characteristics that are similar to those identified by Simone Roach (2002) who carried out an investigation that aimed to clarify the concept of human caring. Roach asked the question 'What is a nurse doing when he or she is caring?' and structured the responses into specific caring behaviours – the six Cs.

- Compassion: making an attempt to experience what the patient is experiencing; taking time to be with the patient.
- Competence: possessing the knowledge and experience for the situation; acquiring factual information, identifying and using relevant knowledge; performing technical procedures to a satisfactory standard.
- Confidence: maintaining trusting relationships; showing respect for patients and their families.
- Conscience: being an advocate for patients; practising patient-centred care; respecting patients' rights; adhering to ethical codes.
- Commitment: supporting patients; putting patients first; demonstrating *a convergence between one's desires and one's obligations, and by a deliberate choice to act in accordance with them* (Roach, 2002, p62).
- Comportment: portraying themselves through their behaviour, with professional, respectful demeanour, bearing, dress and language.

We will now consider some of these caring behaviours in practice, and how they might feature in policy deliberations.

Case study: Ivy, Part 3

During the time Ivy spent in the residential home, her physical condition gradually deteriorated and she became increasingly frail. She started to be reluctant to eat, but could usually be coaxed with her favourite foods. Following an overwhelming and debilitating urinary tract infection, Ivy was admitted to hospital in a very frail state. She was cared for in an acute medical ward, where she refused to get out of bed and also she refused to eat or drink, in spite of every effort being made by the nurses to encourage her. She would clamp her mouth shut at any attempt to get her to eat or drink. By this time her mental state had also deteriorated, and it is doubtful that she knew where she was, though she did have periods of lucidity. One day she said to her daughter They are laughing at me.

Activity 6.4   *Communication*

There are several reasons why Ivy might have perceived that the nurses were laughing at her.

What might these reasons be?

There is a brief outline answer at the end of the chapter.

There is no indication in the case study that the nurses were laughing at Ivy, but this was her perception. Nurses might have been trying to laugh with Ivy; Ivy might have overheard a conversation with another patient; nurses might have been talking to each and sharing a joke as they cared for Ivy. But Ivy's reaction serves as a reminder that nurses need to be careful with their actions and conversations as they are constantly 'on show' and they may easily be misunderstood. This relates particularly to Roach's caring behaviour of comportment, but it also encompasses compassion – something that attracted political attention in 2008 following criticism of the attitudes of some nurses (Sturgeon, 2008). The then Health Secretary, Alan Johnson, announced that nurses were to be scored on how compassionate they were towards patients (Carvel, 2008; Sturgeon, 2008), as part of a plan to improve quality in the NHS. It remains unclear how compassion can be quantified and measured; however, the proposal did prompt much discussion around compassion and also dignity, together with the need to devise metrics in order to be able to produce reliable, quantifiable data about nursing activities.

Case study: Ivy, Part 4

Another time when her family visited, they found Ivy with her bed sheet pulled over her head. When the family members gently pulled back the sheet, Ivy emerged and said to them I didn't say you could come in.

Activity 6.5   *Critical thinking*

Why do you think Ivy had pulled the sheet over her head and then said *I didn't say you could come in?*

There is a brief outline answer at the end of the chapter.

While it is possible that Ivy was confused, her statement is fairly clear. It is quite possible that Ivy was trying to create some private space and exert some control over her life amid the noise and activity of a busy hospital ward. This raises questions of privacy and dignity for any patients, but particularly for older patients in hospital. Privacy is defined as *freedom from unauthorised intrusion* (DH, 2010d, p7). Privacy and dignity are issues that rose to prominence in the early 2000s, following concerns about care for older people.

Privacy and dignity feature in the Essence of Care initiative (DH, 2010e), which provides 12 benchmarks for fundamental aspects of care that are used to support quality improvement. Descriptions of best practice have been developed in partnership with people requiring care and carers. A benchmark is defined as *A standard of best practice and care by which current practice and care is assessed or measured* (DH, 2010e, p9).

Benchmarks for respect and dignity

Benchmarks for respect and dignity are available in the *Essence of Care* document (DH, 2010d). The person-focused outcome for respect and dignity is *People will experience care that is focused on respect* (DH, 2010d, p7). A series of general indicators of best practice are identified, which must be considered alongside specific best practice indicators for seven factors that contribute to the maintenance of respect and dignity. The seven factors are as follows.

1. Attitudes and behaviours.
2. Personal world and personal identity.
3. Personal boundaries and space.
4. Communication.
5. Privacy – confidentiality.
6. Privacy, dignity and modesty.
7. Privacy – private area.
   (DH, 2010d, p8)

An example of a general indicator is: *People feel that care is delivered at all times with compassion and empathy in a respectful and non-judgemental way* (DH, 2010d, p4). An example of a specific indicator of best practice for Factor 6, 'Privacy, dignity and modesty', is: *People are protected from unwanted view, for example, by using curtains, screens, walls, clothes and covers* (DH, 2010d, p16).

There is no shortage of documents and guidance on providing care with compassion, dignity and respect. Nevertheless, lapses in some of the behaviours described by Roach contributed to a series of reports of failings in the NHS amounting to what one newspaper described as *a culture of neglect* in the NHS (Templeton, 2012a). These critical reports also prompted the Prime Minister, David Cameron, to intervene in nursing policy when he made a public announcement calling for NHS hospitals to implement hourly nursing rounds. While politicians regularly pronounce on health policy, it is unusual for them to become involved in nursing policy – though this is not the first time it has happened, as we have already seen that the attention paid to compassion originated with politicians.

The Prime Minister's intervention received varied responses, but his intervention should be seen as an example to nurses of what can happen if the profession does not take control of nursing policy – someone else will. While some people saw the announcement of hourly nursing rounds as a gimmick, the practice draws on 'intentional rounding', which is used in the USA.

Intentional rounding

Intentional rounding involves hourly nursing rounds to check on patients. The National Nursing Research Unit (NNRU, 2012a) reviewed the available evidence relating to intentional rounding and identified the key elements – the '4Ps'.

- Positioning: checking on patients' comfort and pressure ulcer risk assessment.
- Personal needs: for example, taking patients to the bathroom.
- Pain: assessing patients' pain.
- Placement: checking that patients have necessary items within reach.

During each round, as well as checking the 4Ps, nurses are required to engage in other activities, including introducing themselves, performing scheduled tasks and asking patients something on the lines of *Is there anything else I can do for you before I go?* (NNRU, 2012a).

Evidence does suggest that intentional rounding can result in improved outcomes for patients – for example, in relation to more effective pain management and a reduction in the numbers of falls and pressure ulcers (NNRU, 2012a). There are reports of better patient satisfaction, a reduction in complaints, a reduction in the frequency of call-bell usage and a reduction in the length of time patients have to wait for the call bells to be answered (Dix et al., 2012). There are suggestions that time taken to carry out rounds can be offset by savings from improved patient management (NNRU, 2012a).

Dix et al. (2012) describe the former nursing practice of performing regular 'back rounds' in order to reduce the development of pressure ulcers. These rounds were without doubt task oriented, and the imperative of providing individualised and holistic care led to the demise of nursing rounds. However, it is clear that in many cases supposed individual and holistic care is not meeting patients' needs, and intentional rounding appears attractive as a method of re-orienting nursing back to the bedside.

Responses to policy

One response from the Royal College of Nursing and the Royal College of General Practitioners to the unfavourable reports from bodies such as Age Concern (2006, 2010) and the Patients

Association (2011) suggests that relatives should go into hospitals to feed their elderly family members and to take them to the toilet (Templeton, 2011). Many hospitals have encouraged family members to participate in care for some time now; the suggestion from the Royal Colleges did raise questions about whether relatives should feel obliged to engage in these activities. One response pointed to *an indictment of the current state of nursing* (Templeton, 2011, p1), while the Patients Association expressed concern that it could result in nurses absolving themselves from their duty of care.

A more constructive response can be found in the 'Productive Ward' programme, developed by the NHS Institute for Innovation and Improvement.

The Productive Ward programme

The NHS Institute for Innovation and Improvement established the Productive Ward programme as part of its Productive Series, which support NHS staff in shaping management and working practices to improve the quality of care and improve costs (NHS Institute for Innovation and Improvement, 2011). The Productive Ward programme aims to empower ward teams to improve ward processes to help nurses spend more time with patients and make efficiency savings. Improvements for patients and staff have been identified, including better patient experience and staff satisfaction, and reduced harmful events.

The Nursing and Care Quality Forum

This forum was set up by the Prime Minister with the aim of improving the quality of care across all settings. Fundamental elements of good care are identified as compassion, dignity, respect and safety. The Forum is independent and comprises a range of experts on nursing and care, nurses from a range of settings, members of professional bodies, patient representatives and representation from the voluntary sector (Nursing Forum, 2012).

'Friends and Family' test

The Nursing and Care Quality Forum made recommendations in May 2012 which included action to increase the number of staff who would be happy for their friends and family to be treated in their place of work.

The Prime Minister then proposed an NHS 'Friends and Family' test with the aim of improving patient care and identifying the best performing hospitals in England. The test will include a question to be put to all patients in acute inpatient wards and A&E departments about the care they received. The information acquired from the test will be made available to the public to help them make choices about where they would like to be treated.

Caring in the future

There can be no doubt that life expectancy is increasing, which will result in increasing numbers of older people. It is projected that by 2034, 23 per cent of the population will be over the age of 65 years (Parliamentary and Health Service Ombudsman, 2011, p8). There will be more people with multiple and complex health issues, disabilities and long-term conditions. Policy is needed to address this situation at all levels.

Since the early 1990s there has been a politically driven concerted effort to develop the roles of healthcare workers, sometimes blurring traditional professional boundaries (Colyer, 2004). While we have already considered the drive towards more effective collaboration between different professional groups in the name of interprofessional working, one area that we have not yet considered is the important relationship between qualified nurses and healthcare assistants. Recently, developments have been strongly driven by economic considerations. With the prospect of fewer qualified nurses and more healthcare assistants, the role of healthcare assistants has expanded (RCN, 2012b). In the absence of regulation there are no national standards for the education and training of healthcare assistants (RCN, 2012b). The RCN reminds us that registered nurses remain ultimately responsible for the care of their patients and accountable for delegation of caring tasks. However, it has been suggested that supervision of healthcare assistants may be inadequate in some areas (RCN, 2012c) as hospital wards for older people may have a more dilute skill mix than other types of wards. Nurses need time to meet the needs of older people, many of whom have complex care needs. The RCN (2012c) acknowledges that helping someone with swallowing difficulties to eat and drink safely can take thirty minutes or more. Questions have been raised concerning setting minimum levels of staffing to ensure effective care provision. International evidence reviewed by the NNRU (2012b) suggests that there are benefits to nurses attached to setting minimum registered nurse-to-patient ratios, in terms of a more stable workforce and more manageable workloads. However, the impact on patient outcomes is not clear. Setting such ratios has to be specific to specialities and has to take into account local contexts as well as the skill mix (NNRU, 2012b). The RCN has called for regulation of healthcare assistants.

Nursing policy and compassion

In 2012, the NHS Commissioning Board published a consultation document that was written by Jane Cummings, the Chief Nursing Officer for England at the DH, and Viv Bennett, the DH Director for Nursing. The document presents a vision for high-quality compassionate care and invites feedback on the vision and the actions that are identified as necessary for the vision to become reality (NHS Commissioning Board, 2012b; see also www.commissioningboard. nhs.uk/nursingvision/). The document focuses on older people, as they are the biggest group of users of health and social services, and states: *If we can get it right for them, we can also get it right for everyone, including children and young people and other key groups* (NHS Commissioning Board, 2012b, p7). The vision is underpinned by six fundamental values: care, compassion, competence, communication, courage and commitment. These are reminiscent of Roach's six 'C's (Roach, 2002). The consultation represents an example of the nursing profession taking control of nursing policy, and it is also an opportunity for nurses to influence the future of the nursing profession.

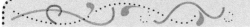

Chapter summary

In this chapter we have seen how reports of poor care have forced caring on to the policy agenda. Greater transparency has resulted in widespread media coverage of these adverse events, which have focused on older people. There are suggestions that these reports do not represent isolated incidents but instead indicate widespread failings within the NHS. While this chapter has highlighted cases of poor care, it is important to note that there are many reports of good care (CQC, 2011a; Parliamentary and Health Service Ombudsman, 2011; Patients Association, 2011). The intention is not to dwell on the revelations of inadequate care but rather to use them to highlight how issues get on to policy agendas. The faults do not lie exclusively with the nursing profession, but the reports do highlight the need for good leadership, and they make recommendations for nursing education. There is evidence of opportunities for nurses to take the lead with improving the quality of care in terms of raising quality to that of best practice. Examples have been provided of what can be achieved when nurses do raise the profile of their good practice. Nurses face challenges in the future as the need for care increases and economic stringency continues.

Activities: Brief outline answers

Activity 6.1: Reflection (page 99)

Your answer will depend on the area you have been working in, but it is likely that many of the carers you have been in contact with are women. You may have encountered male carers of older women; these will usually be husbands. You may also have encountered carers who are in their late middle age who are caring for very old people.

Activity 6.2: Critical thinking (page 100)

All carers are at risk of loss of social life and social isolation. They may experience stress through the sheer volume of caring they have to do, or because they lack the necessary information, knowledge and skills to solve all the problems they encounter. All carers may experience mental and physical health problems. Women in particular are at risk of loss of earnings.

Activity 6.3: Reflection (page 107)

You may have identified characteristics such as being a skilled practitioner; having the ability to meet patients' needs, kindness, caring, being knowledgeable and being conscientious.

Activity 6.4: Communication (page 108)

The nurses may have being trying to joke with Ivy to please her; they may have been laughing with another patient; they may have been sharing a private joke.

Activity 6.5: Critical thinking (page 109)

Ivy may have been confused, but it is possible that she was trying to exert some control over her life and create her own space.

Further reading

Commission on Dignity in Care (2012) *Delivering dignity: securing dignity in care for older people in hospitals and care homes.* Available at: **www.nhsconfed.org/Publications/reports/Pages/Delivering-Dignity.aspx**.

This report contains recommendations for improving dignity in the care of older people.

Dix, G, Phillips, J and Braide, M (2012) Engaging staff with intentional rounding. *Nursing Times*, 108(3): 14–16.

This article describes the implementation of intentional rounding in one hospital, as part of the Back to Basics campaign.

Hall, C and Ritchie, D (2011) *What is nursing? Exploring theory and practice.* Exeter: Learning Matters.

This book explores the real-world role of the nurse in modern healthcare services.

Useful websites

www.cqc.org.uk

The CQC website contains detailed reports on their inspections. As well as reading the findings, it is interesting to read about how the inspections are carried out.

www.ombudsman.org.uk

This website for the Parliamentary and Health Service Ombudsman contains reports of investigations into complaints made to the service.

Chapter 7
Public health policy, inequalities in health and wellbeing and nursing practice

continued . . .

personalised plan that is based on mutual understanding and respect for their individual situation promoting health and well-being, minimising risk of harm and promoting their safety at all times.

Cluster: Infection prevention and control

21. People can trust the newly registered graduate nurse to identify and take effective measures to prevent and control infection in accordance with local and national policy.

By entry to the register:

xi. Recognises infection risk and reports and acts in situations where there is need for health promotion and protection and public health strategies.

Chapter aims

After reading this chapter, you will be able to:

* define public health;
* appreciate the contribution of epidemiology to public health;
* understand the nature and causes of inequalities in health;
* give critical consideration to the implementation of policy that aims to reduce inequalities in health;
* discuss the nurse's role in implementing policy to promote health.

Introduction

Scenario: Ellen

Ellen is 48 years old and has been a hospital nurse for 20 years. Apart from the occasional back trouble she enjoys good health. Whenever she is nursing quite seriously ill women of her own age she thinks This could be me *and wonders what lies behind differences in health and wellbeing.*

This chapter will consider the policies surrounding the public health role of the nurse in relation to protecting people from serious health threats and helping people to live longer, healthier lives. You will consider some of the different health-related measures, such as incidence, prevalence, morbidity, mortality, infant mortality and life expectancy, and their relevance to nursing practice. We will look at social determinants of health and how nurses can help implement policies aimed at reducing inequalities in health and promoting health.

Public health policy

This is a familiar picture. The Department of Health (2011b) warns that 23.1 per cent of 4–5-year-olds and 33.3 per cent of 10–11-year-olds are overweight or obese. Being overweight or obese can lead to type 2 diabetes, heart disease and cancers, and the UK is among the countries with the highest levels of excess weight in the world. The government is concerned because of the cost to the NHS and to the individuals concerned who are likely to have a reduced quality of life. It is not surprising that a concerted effort is being made to reduce the nation's weight (DH, 2011b). The effort entails a cross-government approach to public health with central government aiming to shape an environment that makes it easier for people to adopt and maintain a healthy diet (DH, 2011b).

We will start by considering policy concerning public health. Public health is a concern for all nurses, not just those working in primary care.

Activity 7.1   *Critical thinking*

What do you understand by the term 'public health'?

There is a brief outline answer at the end of the chapter.

The Department of Health (2010f) adopts the following definition of public health from the Faculty of Public Health: *The science and art of preventing disease, prolonging life and promoting health through organised efforts of society* (DH, 2010f, p5).

You will note that the two key elements of public health are the promotion of health and prevention of disease. But you will also note that this modern definition refers to *organised efforts of society*, implying community involvement. Public health policy has its focus 'upstream' (Hunter, 2003), that is, aiming to prevent disease. We will now consider some examples of 'upstream' areas that have been reported in the various media.

Activity 7.2 — *Evidence-based practice and research*

Listen to the news on the television or radio, or have a look at national newspapers.

Look for reports that provide health information to the public and that might have implications for public health.

Is the information provided by the media evidence-based? Is the information correct?

There is a brief outline answer at the end of the chapter.

You may have found a range of topics, including coronary heart disease, mental health, obesity and smoking cessation. Here are a few examples of reports.

- A newspaper article (Sample, 2012) reported on the controversial area of improvements in brain function in children who take omega-3 supplements. The research that was reported also raised controversy as it was conducted independently by Oxford University, but was funded by a company that makes omega-3 supplements. The report suggested that children with very poor reading skills could improve their skills with daily supplements of omega-3.
- A newspaper article (Smithers, 2012) reported on advice from Consensus Action on Salt and Health that bacon is now the second-biggest source of salt in the UK diet after bread.
- A newspaper article (Boseley, 2012) reported on a study published in *The Lancet* medical journal that advised that people in jobs with high demands but little control over decision-making may be at increased risk of heart attacks. This increased risk results from a mismatch between expectations and perceptions, and although the risk spans the entire social spectrum, it is more common in low-income jobs where people are bound by tight schedules over which they have little or no control.

Epidemiology

A broad range of individuals, organisations and disciplines are involved in protecting and improving the health of populations. Epidemiology – the study of patterns of health and illness – has a central role. Public health professionals collect and analyse data about populations in order to acquire epidemiological information about current patterns of health and illness, and also demographic information about their local populations. You will note that while many health professionals focus on their individual patients, the focus of public health is on populations and communities (Baggott, 2000).

Activity 7.3   *Evidence-based practice and research*

Look up the following measures used in epidemiology and make sure you are familiar with them.

- Prevalence.
- Incidence.
- Morbidity.
- Mortality.
- Infant mortality.
- Life expectancy.

There is a brief outline answer at the end of the chapter.

These are just a few of the more basic, and frequently used, measures in epidemiology. Infant mortality and life expectancy are particularly important in that they are often used as indicators of socio-economic progress and development, and are used when comparing countries, as well as different regions of countries. Specific national targets for reducing infant mortality and increasing life expectancy by 2010 were also set by the Labour government in 2001 (Shaw et al., 2005). Reports of trends in, and patterns of, health and illness are frequently made in the media and patients may seek your advice in clarifying what a particular report might mean for them. Familiarity with these measures will form a starting point for you to be able to understand such reports, and to respond to questions from your patients.

Developments in public health

Historically, public health has entailed seeking supplies of clean water and sanitation; a clean water supply and waste disposal are central to development now as in the past. The origins of formal public health in England lie with the public health reformer Edwin Chadwick, who focused his attention on the prevention of infectious diseases, particularly among poor people. Chadwick made the connection between infection and poor sanitation, and his endeavours contributed to the first Public Health Act in 1848, which focused on improving the nation's health through the improvement of sanitation and delivery of clean water (Mason and Whitehead, 2003). Over time, various public health services developed, including sanitation and municipal health services. The creation of the NHS in 1948 consolidated the range of existing services within a national system (Baggott, 2000); however, there were concerns that the NHS was a sickness service rather than a health service. Public health professionals were located in local government until 1974, when a reorganisation of health services integrated public health within the NHS (Hunter, 2003).

Also in 1974 there was an important and influential development when the Minister for Health and Welfare in Canada, Marc Lalonde, drew attention to the limitations of biomedical healthcare systems in improving health and preventing disease. Lalonde's report launched a new era for public health in the Western world, as attention turned towards upstream measures to prevent disease and promote health, and a 'new public health'.

Inequalities in health

Since the 1990s public health policy has been inextricably linked with reducing inequalities in health. While the health of the population as a whole improves, the health of the poorest either improves at a slower pace than the rest of the population or gets worse (Graham and Kelly, 2004). This suggests that some policy works, but it fails the poorest (Graham and Kelly, 2004).

Although awareness of health inequalities in Britain has existed since the 1850s (Macintyre, 1997), the defining point of awareness in Britain was probably the publication of the Black Report in 1980 (Townsend et al., 1992). A working group was set up by the Secretary of State for Health to investigate variations in the health and illness experience of different groups of people following his recognition that:

> *the crude differences in mortality rates between the various social classes are worrying . . . in 1971 the death rate for adult men in social class V (unskilled workers) was nearly twice that of adult men in social class I (professional workers . . .)*
> (Townsend et al., 1992, p1)

Particularly worrying at the time was the fact that this awareness of differences in mortality rates existed against the background of a National Health Service that was set up with the express intention of treating people equitably. The working group completed its review of evidence in 1980 and concluded that the poorer health experience of the lower occupational group, previously identified in relation to adult men, applied to both men and women at all stages of life (Townsend et al., 1992).

At the time the working group did acknowledge difficulty in identifying exactly how poverty and the class structure cause ill health and death, but it argued strongly that a key concept linking higher mortality rates with social class was material deprivation. These inequalities in mortality rates were not necessarily a function of the NHS, though it did appear that middle-class patients had longer consultations with their doctors than working-class patients and that they were able to make better use of that consultation time (Townsend et al., 1992). More recently, Goddard and Smith (2001) identified that higher rates of GP consultation are associated with greater deprivation and with lower socio-economic groups, though manual groups continued to be less likely to consult GPs for preventative care than those in higher social classes.

Scenario: Albert

Albert is a 74-year-old retired merchant seaman. He lives with his wife in accommodation that is rented from a Housing Association. Albert and his wife enjoy life, particularly their weekly evening at the local social club with friends and neighbours. Albert also has an allotment and grows some vegetables.

Albert went to see his GP because he had some abdominal discomfort and rectal bleeding. He didn't want to go to the GP, but his wife persuaded him that he should. The GP referred him to a gastro-intestinal surgeon who saw Albert in his outpatient department clinic and decided to admit him soon to hospital for investigations

continued . . .

under general anaesthetic. The nurse in the outpatient clinic explained to Albert that he would have to be starved prior to the examinations and that he would have to have bowel preparation.

Albert went home and thought about the impending investigations – he did not like the sound of them at all. Albert was frightened, as he had read in his newspaper about elderly people being starved in hospital and losing weight. For example, a newspaper article (Templeton, 2012b) described how an elderly woman died in hospital after she was left weakened by repeatedly being denied water while waiting for surgery. He had also heard about older people being put on the Liverpool Care Pathway, being denied food and drink, and not being given active treatment. Besides, he was feeling better and just wanted to get back to his allotment.

Albert is considering not going into hospital for investigations.

People in different socio-economic groups have different health experiences, and these are related to occupation, income and education. These experiences can be seen in terms of mortality and morbidity – for example, professional households report less long-term illness than unskilled manual households (Baggott, 2004). Albert's scenario provides an example of a man who is fearful of going into hospital and having further investigations. This fear may be well founded, but a person with a more professional background might spend time finding out more about the investigations and possible outcomes, more about the surgeon's own expertise and research profile, and more about the performance record of the hospital they are going to attend. Albert lacks the resources to explore the proposed investigations and the confidence to find answers to his questions.

Activity 7.4   Communication

How would you help Albert to reconsider his approach to the impending investigations?

There is a brief outline answer at the end of the chapter.

While all patients should be given similar information, more 'informed' patients might demand more and have more questions to ask. The nurse's contribution to reducing inequalities in health is to ensure that patients asking fewer questions have all the information that is necessary for them to make informed decisions. Later in this chapter we will come across the principle of 'proportionate universalism'.

The Black Report made many recommendations for policies that would help to reduce inequalities in health, but the government of the day was not convinced that the evidence satisfactorily supported the recommendations. Consequently, the recommendations – which related largely to socio-economic interventions – were not fully implemented. However, the interest aroused by the findings of the Black Report prompted volumes of research into inequalities in health and several reports commissioned by governments.

Inequalities in health between rich and poor areas of Britain continued to widen in the 1980s and 1990s (Shaw et al., 2005). The Labour party came to power in 1997 and published a Green

Paper with a commitment to tackling inequalities in health (DH, 1998b). It had two aims: to improve life expectancy and the number of years people spend free from illness; and to improve the health of the worst off in society and thus narrow the health gap between richest and poorest. This was also the first government that explicitly acknowledged the contribution of socio-economic factors to ill health. Successive Labour governments went on to attempt to reduce inequalities in health – which mirror inequalities in income – by addressing some of the socio-economic factors that play a part. Their policies were influenced by the Acheson Report (Acheson, 1998), which reviewed evidence on inequalities in health and informed policy development for the following ten years. The Acheson Report highlighted the widening gap between social groups and recommended policy responses, which included tackling poverty and introducing initiatives and programmes to encourage cross-sector partnerships.

While inequalities in health had mostly been explained by health-related behaviour and material deprivation, Wilkinson's (1992, 1996) work highlighted a further factor, arguing that the social consequences of people's differing circumstances in terms of stress, self-esteem and social relations may now be one of the most important influences on health.

Inequalities of health at the international level

Policy relating to inequalities in health exists at the international level. We saw in Chapter 1 how the WHO is influential in policy relating to promoting health. The WHO Regional Office for Europe (2012) notes that it makes sense to invest in health; good health has benefits for society. Health 2020 is the new health policy framework of the WHO European region and proposes 'Health in all Policies' through cross-government working with other departments, as well as with wider society. The goal is to:

> *significantly improve the health and wellbeing of populations, reduce health inequalities, strengthen public health and ensure people-centred health systems that are universal, equitable, sustainable and of high quality.*
> (WHO Regional Office for Europe, 2012, p1)

An important WHO publication in terms of shaping health policy in the UK came from the Commission on Social Determinants of Health.

Social determinants of health

The Commission on Social Determinants of Health (CSDH, 2008) was established in order to consider the evidence on actions to promote equity in health and to promote a global approach to reducing inequalities in health.

Activity 7.5 *Evidence-based practice and research*

What are 'social determinants of health'?

Search in your university library for 'social determinants of health', or visit the following websites in order to answer the question.

---

continued . . .

* www.instituteofhealthequity.org
* www.who.int/social_determinants/thecommission/finalreport/en/index.html.
Commission on Social Determinants of Health (CSDH, 2008) *Closing the gap in a generation: health equity through action on the social determinants of health*. Geneva: WHO. You should be able to watch a short video of an interview with Professor Sir Michael Marmot by clicking on the link.

There is a brief outline answer at the end of the chapter.

As a nurse you will need to understand the social determinants of health as this work is paramount in informing current health policy. You will have found that social determinants of health are the *conditions in which people are born, grow, live, work and age . . .* (CSDH, 2008). These include social position, education, occupation, income, gender, ethnicity/race – all of which can have an impact on an individual's material circumstances, social cohesion, psychosocial factors, behaviours and biological factors (CSDH, 2008).

According to the CSDH, action on the social determinants of health must involve the whole of government and all sectors of society. Three principles of action have been identified.

* Improve the conditions of daily life – the circumstances in which people are born, grow, live, work and age.
* Tackle the inequitable distribution of power, money and resources – the structural drivers of those conditions of daily life – globally, nationally and locally.
* Measure the problem, evaluate action, expand the knowledge base, develop a workforce that is trained in the social determinants of health and raise public awareness about the social determinants of health (CSDH, 2008).

While most of the responsibility lies with governments, there are areas in the above three principles of action where nurses can make a difference. These are some examples.

* Helping to give children a better start in life.
* Helping with healthy ageing through work with older people.
* Helping to reduce unequal power distributions by educating people about health.
* Engaging in, and publishing, good-quality, robust research in order to understand inequalities in health. We will return to the role of research in Chapter 8.

We will now look at examples of contributions that nurses have made to reducing health inequalities in health. The following is an example of nurses engaging in a programme to help young mothers that has a strong evidence base.

Research summary: The Family Nurse Partnership Programme

The Family Nurse Partnership Programme (FNP) is an intervention programme for vulnerable young first-time mothers that can form part of NHS and local authority joint strategies for children. There are 74 FNP teams in 80 local areas in England. The FNP programme aims to:

- improve pregnancy outcomes;
- improve child health and development;
- improve parents' economic self-sufficiency.

All first-time mothers aged 19 and under at conception are eligible, and participation in the programme is voluntary. The programme consists of intensive and structured home visiting, provided by specially trained nurses, from early pregnancy until the child is aged two years, when families are transferred to health visiting services so that the remainder of the Healthy Child programme can be completed.

The FNP programme has a strong evidence base of benefits to families in need in the USA. The original work in the USA found that FNP resulted in improved outcomes when delivered by highly qualified nurses. The strength of the nursing contribution lies in trust in and respect for the nursing profession as well as the academic preparation in social, life and caring sciences.

There is a strong theoretical base to the programme. Nurses use theory and expertise to engage in behaviour change methods to foster adoption of healthier lifestyles by the families. While nurses have guidelines to follow, they also have sufficient autonomy to use their professional judgement to address areas where needs are greatest. You can find more information at the end of the chapter.

The next example entails nurse-led projects to widen access to hospice services.

Case study: *Towards excellence in hospice care: widening access through nurse leadership*

Help the Hospices is a charity, and has been working to develop equitable hospice care. Categories of disadvantage in relation to access to end-of-life care and hospice services include the oldest members of society; people from black and minority ethnic groups; gay and lesbian people; people with learning disabilities and mental health needs; people with dementia; and residents of care homes and prisons (Help the Hospices, 2012). Further, most people who use hospice services have cancer; there are many people with long-term conditions such as heart failure and chronic obstructive pulmonary disease who are not able to access hospice services.

Amid these concerns, Help the Hospices has developed a nurse leadership programme to widen access to hospice services. The charity supports innovative nurse-led projects that aim to enhance leadership abilities while at the

continued . . .

same time making a positive impact on widening access to hospice services. Examples of the nurse-led projects include:

- *developing outreach services – holding weekly clinics in GP centres to enable more people to be seen nearer to home;*
- *rural support for isolated patients and their carers – members of the multidisciplinary hospice team provide a programme for carers;*
- *transition of care – working across organisational boundaries to improve the transition from long-term care to palliative care.*

Inequalities in health at national level

A further review of inequalities in health in England was commissioned by the Secretary of State for Health in 2008. The Marmot Review was published in 2010 and concluded that people in higher socio-economic positions have more life chances and better health, consolidating the link between social conditions and health. While on the whole people in England are living longer than before, variations in health are found across England. People living in disadvantaged areas are more likely to have a shorter life expectancy and worse health than those living in more advantaged areas (Marmot Review, 2010).

However, inequalities do not imply a simple relationship between the richest and poorest: there is a social gradient in health. There is now widespread acknowledgement that there is a step-wise gradient in health, and this is supported by the findings of the Whitehall studies (Marmot, 1996; Bosma et al., 1997; Marmot and Davey Smith, 1997) and the research base that relates disease patterns to the organisation of society (Marmot, 1999). The Marmot Review (2010) recommends that action should focus on reducing the gradient. Action to address health inequalities requires action to address the social determinants of health: *To reduce the steepness of the social gradient in health, actions must be universal, but with a scale and intensity that is proportionate to the level of disadvantage. We call this proportionate universalism* (Marmot Review, 2010, p9).

Research summary: The Jubilee line of health inequality

The title of this research refers to the Jubilee line of the London Underground, which runs from Stanmore to Stratford. Using data from 2004 to 2008, the London Health Observatory has identified differences in male life expectancy within a small area of London – the so called 'Jubilee line of health inequality' (London Health Observatory, 2010). Travelling from west to east along the Jubilee line from Westminster, every two tube stations represent over one year of life expectancy lost.

Health inequalities exist in relation to social class, ethnicity, gender and ability. However, it is important to remember that inequalities can interact and individuals may have multiple identities. For example, an Asian man might also have mental health problems, which could affect his ability to retain a job, and so have an impact on his socio-economic status.

Ethnicity and health

At the time of the Black Report 'race' had rarely been assessed in official censuses and surveys in Britain (Townsend et al., 1992). It was also not clear which indicator should be used when investigating health – 'race' or ethnicity (Townsend et al., 1992). Researchers utilised varying indicators – for example, mortality rates relating to country of birth of the deceased (Balarajan and Soni Raleigh, 1993) and country of family origin (Nazroo, 1997). Census data concerning ethnicity is now available.

One early and important study (Balarajan and Soni Raleigh, 1993) identified the biggest difference in health and illness in relation to coronary heart disease (CHD), with mortality from CHD being higher among people born in the Indian subcontinent than among the white majority population in Britain and also other minority ethnic groups. However, later studies (Balarajan, 1996; Bhopal et al., 1999) showed that grouping disparate ethnic groups under one heading can be misleading. When people born in the Indian sub-continent were identified in separate groupings, it was found that mortality in CHD was highest among Bangladeshis, followed by Pakistanis and then Indians. There is a tendency for Indians to enjoy a better socio-economic profile than Pakistanis and Bangladeshis, leading Balarajan (1996) to suggest social class as a mediating factor among the determinants of CHD. Factors relating to socio-economic status are therefore important when considering ethnic health in Britain. People from minority ethnic groups are likely to experience poverty and disadvantage, as identified by higher unemployment rates, a greater reliance on social housing, lower incomes and lower car ownership, which, together with racism, may affect their health (HEA, 1994; Smaje, 1995; Nazroo, 1998).

Social justice

Some determinants of health, such as age, race and gender, cannot be changed. However, many inequalities in health are avoidable and this is a matter of social justice (Marmot Review, 2010).

Concept summary: social justice

It is difficult to define the notion of social justice in a few words. The Commission on Social Justice (1994) identified four principles of social justice.

- Equal worth of all citizens.
- Equal right to be able to meet basic needs.
- Need to spread opportunities and life chances as widely as possible.
- Requirement to reduce and where possible eliminate unjustified inequalities.
  (Burchardt and Craig, 2008, p1)

A strategy for public health

The Coalition government responded to the report on social determinants in health *Fair society, healthy lives* (Marmot Review, 2010) and adopted its life course framework for tackling the wider social determinants of health. The Coalition government eschews targets in favour of outcomes and relocates control of public health from central to local government by empowering local government and local communities to reduce inequalities and improve health at key stages in people's lives.

The White Paper for public health in England *Healthy lives, healthy people: our strategy for public health in England* (DH, 2010f) is about empowering people to make healthy choices. The approach to improving health and wellbeing reflects the Coalition's core values of freedom, fairness and responsibility.

- Strengthening self-esteem, confidence and personal responsibility.
- Positively promoting 'healthier' behaviours and lifestyles.
- Adapting the environment to make healthy choices easier.
 (DH, 2010f, p29)

The aim is thus to make the healthier choice the easier choice, and this is an idea expressed by Thaler and Sunstein (2009) in their influential book *Nudge*.

Concept summary: Nudge

Nudge is an idea articulated in the USA. The idea involves employing the services of a 'choice architect' who organises an environment in which people make decisions, with the intention of focusing people's attention in a particular direction. For example, if there is a desire to have an impact on people's behaviour relating to healthy eating, the 'choice architect' might place healthier food such as fruit at eye level. The aim is to influence people's behaviour in order to make their lives longer, healthier and better. The underpinning principles include preserving freedom of choice while at the same time 'nudging' people in directions that will improve their lives (Thaler and Sunstein, 2009).

Organisational changes are necessary in order to effect the changes announced in the White Paper. Responsibilities for local health improvement will transfer from Primary Care Trusts to local authorities. Directors of Public Health will be the strategic leaders for public health and health inequalities in local communities, working in partnership with the local NHS and across the public, private and voluntary sectors. A new professional public health service Public Health England will take over the functions of Health Protection Agency and will support local inter-sectoral innovation.

The approach to addressing the causes of poor health will be:

- responsive – owned by communities and shaped by their needs;
- resourced – with ring-fenced funding and incentives to improve;

- rigorous – professionally led, focused on evidence, efficient and effective; and
- resilient – strengthening protection against current and future threats to health.
  (DH, 2010f, p6)

Wellbeing

You will probably have noticed that the term 'wellbeing' has entered the language of health policy, to the extent that the Coalition government adopted wellbeing in its document *Our health and wellbeing today* (DH 2010g), which accompanied the Public Health White Paper.

Activity 7.6   *Reflection*

What do you understand by the term 'wellbeing'?

What is the relationship between 'health' and 'wellbeing'?

There is a brief outline answer at the end of the chapter.

Concept summary: Wellbeing

The success of individual countries used to be measured only by economic growth. The former president of France, Nicolas Sarkozy, was dissatisfied with this and helped establish the Commission on the Measurement of Economic Performance and Social Progress, which was led by a leading economist. The report (Stiglitz et al., 2009) described a gap between statistical measurements of socio-economic factors and citizen perceptions of these factors, and argued that commonly used measures might not capture some factors that have an impact on the wellbeing of citizens.

For example, the Commission identified several dimensions of wellbeing: material living standards; health; education; personal activities including work; political voice and governance; social connections and relationships; environment; and insecurity, of an economic as well as a physical nature (Stiglitz et al., 2009, p15). The report suggests a shift of emphasis *from measuring economic production to measuring people's well-being* (Stiglitz et al., 2009, p12).

You can see that health is a part of wellbeing and wellbeing is a broad concept that embraces the cross-government approach to improving health that we are currently experiencing. Wellbeing is also being measured in England. The document *Our health and wellbeing today* (DH, 2010g) is a review of the evidence on the health and wellbeing of people in England. It has informed the government's new approach and proposed outcomes framework for public health; it adopts a life course approach to health and wellbeing (p3).

- Starting well – checking the health of mothers pre- and during pregnancy and encouraging good parenting.
- Developing well – encouraging healthy habits in children.

- Growing up well – avoiding/recognising and treating mental health problems in childhood.
- Living and working well – developing good lifestyle choices in adulthood.
- Ageing well – supporting older people to remain resilient to ill health – social networks and protection of vulnerable people.

The document adopts broad definitions of health and wellbeing, and recognises the value of the contribution of healthy people to society, noting that poor health places a strain on individuals, the NHS, the economy and society. The major causes of mortality in England are still CHD, cancers and respiratory diseases. Concern is expressed that the number of people with long-term conditions will rise: people are living longer. Life expectancy for men is 78 years and for women it is 82 years (DH, 2010g, p7). However, longer life is not necessarily spent in good health. So the government now considers quality of life as well as length of life. It is predicted that there will be an increase in age-related conditions such as diabetes, dementia and arthritis.

Mental health

In recognition of the scale of mental health problems, the government gives a high priority in the document (DH, 2010g) to improving mental health. This attention is welcomed by the Royal College of Psychiatrists, which estimates that 22.8 per cent of the total burden of disease in the UK could be attributed to mental illness in 2004 (Royal College of Psychiatrists, 2010, p11), making mental illness the largest single source of illness in the UK. Mental illness is associated with social exclusion and all that it entails, and has huge human and economic consequences. As most mental illnesses have their origins before adulthood, there is a strong case for promoting mental health and preventing mental illness through cross-government activity.

Scenario: Alice

Alice is 11 years old and has been unhappy since her mother died of breast cancer one year ago. Alice is exhibiting emotional problems that have resulted in her being withdrawn at school. She has also been bullied at school. The school nurse has talked with Alice's father, and Alice is now having counselling.

The Coalition government has reaffirmed its commitment to improving mental health and wellbeing with the publication *No health without mental health: implementation framework* (Her Majesty's Government, 2012b). This framework translates the vision of improving mental health and wellbeing into action, claiming that improvements in mental health and wellbeing can contribute to the achievement of the broader aims of improving outcomes across health and social care. The implementation framework has six objectives.

- More people will have good mental health.
- More people with mental health problems will recover.
- More people with mental health problems will have good physical health.
- More people will have a positive experience of care and support.

- Fewer people will suffer avoidable harm.
- Fewer people will experience stigma and discrimination.
  (Her Majesty's Government, 2012b, p8)

Actions are suggested for several organisations and agencies, including commissioners of care, service providers, local authorities, community groups, employers, the criminal justice system and housing organisations. Actions range from support and treatment through to tackling stigma in society.

Multicultural UK

Migrants made up approximately 12 per cent of the UK population in 2010, and most migrants are young people seeking to study or work in the UK (HPA, 2011). The Health Protection Agency (HPA) claims that a small proportion of migrants bear the greatest burden of infectious disease reported in the UK. For example, 73 per cent of reported cases of tuberculosis in the UK were in people who were born abroad (HPA, 2011; NICE, 2012). However, it is important not to view migrants as 'importers of disease', as 77 per cent of these cases were diagnosed two or more years after arrival in the UK (HPA, 2011). This suggests that living conditions in the UK may contribute to this burden of disease.

Cultural competence

Against the background of Europe's increasing diversity The Council of Europe issued a White Paper on intercultural dialogue (Council of Europe, 2010):

> *Intercultural dialogue (ID) is understood as an open and respectful exchange of views between individuals, groups with different ethnic, cultural, religious and linguistic backgrounds and heritage on the basis of mutual understanding and respect. It operates at all levels – within societies, between the societies of Europe and between Europe and the wider world.*
> (Council of Europe, 2010, p14)

The ideas contained in the document are based on individual human dignity and aim to prevent ethnic, religious, linguistic and cultural divides, noting that while diversity can promote creativity, inequalities can create conflicts. The White Paper states that intercultural competences should be taught and learned. Further, training nurses in cultural competence plays an important part of assuring access to health services for all members of the community (ICN, 2011).

Several models exist to assist with the development of cultural competence. One such model is the Papadopoulos, Tilki and Taylor (PTT) model (Papadopoulos, 2006) – see Figure 7.1.

The model proceeds through four main constructs. The first construct is cultural awareness. It is very important that nurses are aware of the importance of culture in determining beliefs about health and illness, and in shaping responses to health and illness. The best way to develop cultural awareness is by thinking about your own culture and how it influences your health behaviours. Then you can start to appreciate how important culture is in relation to your patients' health and illness experiences. Cultural awareness is followed by cultural knowledge. These two constructs set the foundation for the development of cultural sensitivity, and eventually nurses can progress

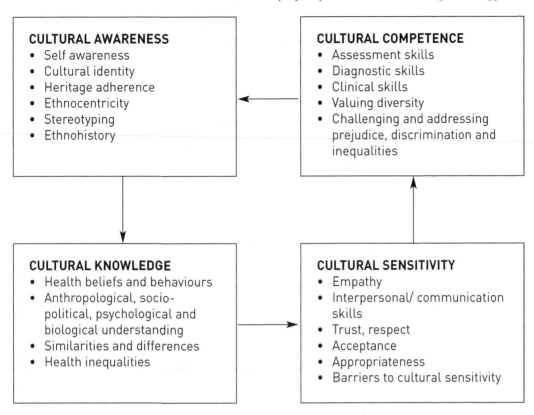

Figure 7.1 The PTT model for developing cultural competence

Source: This model was published in Papadopoulos, I (ed.) *Transcultural health and social care: development of culturally competent practitioners*, p10. London: Elsevier. Copyright Elsevier, 2006.

to cultural competence. However, cultural competence is not an end-point but a continuous process as part of life-long learning as society becomes increasingly diverse. Cultural knowledge entails learning about the health beliefs and behaviours of particular groups of patients, but this is becoming increasingly difficult as the population becomes increasingly diverse. Lipson and DeSantis (2007) report that while the tendency to learn 'cultural characteristics' has a place in nursing, such an approach can foster stereotyping; these authors favour developing the skills to negotiate culturally sensitive care with patients. We will now look at an example of the need for nurses to work towards cultural competence as they implement policy in relation to reducing inequalities in health.

Tuberculosis

Tuberculosis (TB) is stigmatised in many cultures, and this may prevent people seeking help. Such stigma can act as a barrier to early diagnosis and adherence to prescribed treatment for tuberculosis. Stigma is intersubjective, in that it arises from a perceived threat to the stigmatiser and compounds the suffering of the stigmatised (Yang et al., 2007).

> **Research summary: perception and social consequences of tuberculosis**
>
> Following focus group discussions with patients who were hospitalised with TB in Pakistan, Liefooghe et al. (1995) found that TB was viewed as a family disease and that a diagnosis of TB caused distress among family members and could result in the entire family being shunned. For the individual sufferer, anger at the diagnostic label could lead to rejection of the diagnosis of TB or requests that the diagnosis of TB should not be revealed to relatives and neighbours. A diagnosis of TB could have adverse effects on marriage prospects for women sufferers.

You will now consider this case study.

Case study: a Somali community in London

There are concerns at a local health centre that a local Somali community might be at risk of developing tuberculosis and might not have the necessary knowledge to recognise the symptoms and take appropriate action. There are also concerns that there might be reluctance within the community to approach healthcare professionals.

A small of team of nurses and a health visitor have engaged the assistance of a respected leader within the Somali community and are working together with the community to raise awareness about tuberculosis. However, there are some obstacles to overcome as an initial response from the community is Why are you picking on us?

Awareness that TB is stigmatised in many communities might have prompted the nurses to gain more knowledge about the Somali community. This could have been achieved by talking with the community leader – this is usually someone who is respected within the community and often has a professional background. Many community leaders are healthcare professionals, teachers or lawyers who are not allowed to practise their profession in the UK. These community leaders usually speak good English and so are able to represent the community and negotiate with the various services that might be available to the community. Community leaders also function as 'gatekeepers' to the community. With some awareness and knowledge about the community, the nurses could then use their interpersonal and communication skills to negotiate with the community to engage in activities to raise awareness about TB.

There has been a steady increase in the incidence of TB in the UK since the late 1980s, but the incidence varies in different parts of England and Wales; it is particularly high in London.

Policy and TB

NICE public health guidance *Identifying and managing tuberculosis among hard-to-reach groups* (NICE, 2012) provides guidance in relation to people who may be made 'hard to reach' by social circumstances, language, culture or lifestyle. The main groups considered in the guidance are people who are homeless, substance misusers, prisoners and vulnerable migrants.

The document states that the recommendations will be of benefit to the wider community by helping to reduce the spread of TB in the general population as well as preventing and treating TB among the groups identified. The guidance has implications for nurses as it includes specialist TB nurses whose role includes ensuring that TB services are effective; nurse-led clinics to improve access for hard-to-reach groups; and outreach services in convenient locations.

NICE guidelines on the diagnosis and management of TB state that treatment for non-drug-resistant TB entails a six-month course of multiple antibiotics, while the course of treatment for people with the drug-resistant strain lasts for 18 months or longer (NICE, 2011). It is not surprising, therefore, that there are concerns that affected individuals may not adhere to their drug regimes with consequences for their own health and wider public health. The guidelines stress that treatment and care, and the information people are given, should be culturally appropriate.

Chapter summary

The International Council of Nurses (ICN) asserts that *nurses are essential to improving equity and access to health care and adding quality to the outcome of care* (ICN, 2011, p1). This chapter has introduced the key principles of the Coalition government's agenda for public health. There are themes of collaborative working within government, with the NHS and with communities in order to improve population health. Inequalities in health are a feature of life in the UK – many of these inequalities are avoidable. Examples of how nurses can contribute to a reduction in inequalities in health have been given.

Activities: Brief outline answers

Activity 7.1: Critical thinking (page 117)

You might have thought about health promotion and disease prevention, and the health of populations.

Activity 7.2: Evidence-based practice and research (page 118)

There is no shortage of media reports that provide information about health. It is important for nurses to be able to assess the information that is provided in terms of its reliability and credibility. For example, is the information based on research? If so, is the research of good quality? Is the evidence sound? Is the information provided correct? You will need to use your knowledge of research methods to assess whether or not the information has acquired through a rigorous research process.

Activity 7.3: Evidence-based practice and research (page 119)

Prevalence	the number of cases of a disease in a population in a given period of time.
Incidence	the number of *new* cases of a disease in a population in a given period of time.
Morbidity	ill health; for example, morbidity data might include cancer registrations and notifiable diseases.
Mortality	data on deaths.

Infant mortality   the number of deaths in children under one year of age.

Life expectancy   the number of years an individual can be expected to live.

Activity 7.4: Communication (page 121)

You could invite Albert to attend a pre-admission clinic where you could sit with him in a quiet area and explain in detail the nature of the investigations and the reasons for starving prior to the investigations and the bowel preparation. Albert should be given clear information about how long before the procedure he would be required to stop eating and drinking. He should also be told what he can expect following the procedure. Albert should be invited to ask questions.

Activity 7.5: Evidence-based practice and research (pages 122–3)

You will have found that the social determinants of health include people's living and working conditions, and their lifestyles.

Activity 7.6: Reflection (page 128)

Health is generally thought of as part of wellbeing, which is a broader concept.

Further reading

Baggott, R (2010) *Public health: policy and politics* (2nd edn). Basingstoke: Palgrave Macmillan.

This book includes a historical introduction to public health and a detailed account of policies and services.

DH (2012) The Family Nurse Partnership Programme. Information leaflet. Available at: **www.dh.gov. uk/health/2012/07/family-nurse-partnership-programme-information-leaflet/**.

This leaflet gives more information on the Family Nurse Partnership programme. See also the USA website **www.nursefamilypartnership.org**.

Evans, D, Coutsaftiki, D and Fathers, CP (2011) *Health promotion and public health for nursing students.* Exeter: Learning Matters.

This book takes a topical approach to the theory and practice of health promotion and public health.

Marmot, M (2004) *Status syndrome: how your social standing directly affects your health and life expectancy.* London: Bloomsbury.

Wilkinson, R and Pickett, K (2009) *The spirit level: why more equal societies almost always do better.* London: Allen Lane.

Both of the above titles give further information concerning psychosocial stress as a contributor to inequalities in health.

Pless-Mulloli, T, Unwin, N and Carr, S (2007) *An introductory guide to public health and epidemiology* (2nd edn). Buckingham: Open University Press.

This book provides an accessible introduction to epidemiology.

Useful websites

www.instituteofhealthequity.org

This website provides a wealth of information and reports on aspects of inequalities in health.

www.who.int/social_determinants/en/

This website provides more information on global social determinants of health.

Chapter 8
Using policy in nursing practice

Chapter aims

After reading this chapter, you will be able to:

- engage in policy-related discussions with colleagues;
- give consideration to your own policy awareness;
- enhance your knowledge of policy;
- give critical consideration to policy implementation;
- reflect on opportunities to influence policy.

Introduction

Scenario: Pranav

Pranav has been working as a mental health nurse for nearly 20 years. He has seen policy implemented well on his unit, but also times when it is not. He often wonders whether the policy makers would be interested in learning from his experience, and if not, why this is.

This chapter consolidates the content of previous chapters and provides the opportunity for you to look to the future in terms of developing your own policy awareness and your role in implementing policy in practice. In this final chapter we will look at the four 'policy levels': policy awareness, policy knowledge, implementing policy and influencing policy.

There can be no doubt that nurses are working in challenging times: the NHS needs to make savings of £20 billion by 2014/15, and the healthcare environment is becoming increasingly complex and uncertain. The NHS is undergoing momentous change as a result of the Health and Social Care Act 2012. The UK is home to a very diverse population, giving rise to a 'super-diversity' that challenges traditional multicultural models (Phillimore, 2010). The Royal College of Physicians (RCP), in its report *Hospitals on the edge? The time for action* (RCP, 2012b), warns that the NHS is not equipped to deal with the rising number of patients with multiple complex needs, including dementia. The report describes how there are fewer beds available but increasing numbers of emergency admissions. In addition, 65 per cent of patients admitted to hospital are over 65 years. Furthermore, the economic downturn since 2008 may be taking its toll on people's health. A survey of 300 GPs across the UK indicates that people's stress levels are raised because of money worries and having to work longer hours (Insight Research Group, 2012). It is important to understand what the policies mean for nursing practice against this complex and uncertain background accompanied by a raft of new policies. We have seen how policy initiated at the international level – for example, by the WHO or EU – can influence national policy, which in turn is translated into local policy. Policies are also made locally at NHS trust or ward/department level. It has been argued that opportunities arise for nurses to influence policy making, but in order to be in a position to do so they need to develop policy awareness.

Policy awareness

While policy may seem remote from the day-to-day practice of nursing, it does shape how you carry out your work. When you listen to the news on television or radio, or read national or local newspapers or nursing journals, you will often find reports on aspects of health and healthcare policy. For example, on 27 September 2012 Sir David Nicholson, the Chief Executive of the NHS, appeared on national television news to inform the viewing public that the NHS is on 'high alert' to make sure there are no failings, as it prepares for the reorganisation that will take effect from April 2013, and is described as the biggest change since its creation (Jeffreys and Triggle, 2012).

Activity 8.1   *Critical thinking*

Think about your current or recent clinical placement. Why do you think it is necessary for nurses to have policy awareness in that area of practice?

There is a brief outline answer at the end of the chapter.

Your answer will depend to an extent on your chosen area of practice, but key themes running through current health and healthcare policy that apply to all areas of practice are those of quality and safety. You might have thought of policies relating to the special nature of your area of practice – for example, there are NSFs and NICE guidelines and standards for a range of conditions, as well as outcomes that have to be met. On the other hand, you might have thought of policies that are forcing efficiency savings to be made in your area of practice. Being aware of policy is the first step, but in order to be able to use the policy, you have to be knowledgeable about it.

Policy knowledge

Appropriate knowledge is necessary in order to influence policy (Antrobus, 2003). Nurses tend to be 'invisible' in policy debates and lack confidence to enter the policy arena (Fyffe, 2009). Nurses tend to implement policy, but can sometimes experience conflict when policy imperatives are not congruent with nursing values (Daly et al., 2004). For example, at Mid Staffordshire NHS Trust the emphasis on meeting policy-driven targets detracted from quality of care. Nurses may be reluctant to engage in policy discussions because of a fear of conflict (Antrobus, 2003); after all, policy making can entail listening to competing arguments from different stakeholders. Daly et al. (2004, p17) argue that nurses *need to overcome their insecurities and raise controversial issues in a way that encourages discussion.*

Activity 8.2   *Decision-making*

In order to improve your policy awareness, knowledge and confidence in putting across a point of view, gather together a group of your colleagues and organise a debate. A debate allows participants to present an argument, having first read appropriate material and considered two opposing views.

Here are two examples:

• 'The state should be responsible for a nation's health.'
• 'Today's sick people will always take priority over tomorrow's potentially sick people, so moving money from acute healthcare services to health promotion is wrong.'

You need: a chairperson; two people to speak for the motion; two people to speak against the motion; and an audience. The chairperson sets the rules for the debate and introduces the topic. The first proposer presents the motion, followed by the first opposer of the motion. The second proposer speaks and is then followed by the second opposer. A discussion then follows.

There is no answer for this activity. Your discussion will be based on beliefs and opinions and thus there is no right or wrong answer. The activity is an opportunity to practise putting your point of view across.

You will no doubt have expressed some differences of opinion, and your arguments may have drawn on ethical issues. The following case study concerns health policy for asylum seekers whose application for refugee status in the UK has been rejected – otherwise known as 'failed' asylum seekers. The case study shows how doctors used ethical principles to oppose government policy that aimed to deny failed asylum seekers access to free treatment from GPs.

Case study: access to free treatment for failed asylum seekers

In 2008 the Department of Health planned to withdraw from failed asylum seekers the right to free GP treatment. Resistance among GPs to these plans forced ministers to consider abandoning the plans (Hinsliff, 2008a). While the plans proposed that overseas visitors would be eligible for free GP treatment only in emergency situations or for the treatment of selected communicable diseases, including tuberculosis, concerns were raised by GPs that the proposals could contribute to the spread of communicable diseases such as measles and diphtheria if access to vaccinations was denied (Hinsliff, 2008b). There was also a risk that failed asylum seekers, denied treatment by GPs, might go instead to A&E departments, or wait until their illnesses were advanced before seeking treatment as emergencies. Under the plans, asylum seekers whose claims were unsuccessful would be forced to pay for private care or go without. While official guidelines stated that GPs should not register failed asylum seekers, GPs retained the right to use their own discretion. Many GPs threatened to defy government policy, claiming that they would be failing in their duty if they did not treat failed asylum seekers: the practice would be unethical (Hinsliff, 2008a).

The Department of Health was forced to consider abandoning the plans in the light of pressure from doctors.

This is a clear example of how a powerful group of professionals can influence policy by using their knowledge of the proposed policy and their knowledge of ethical principles. It could also be argued that to deny such a vulnerable group of people access to free treatment from GPs was unfair or unjust.

Concept summary: Rawls' theory of social justice

One well-known theory of social justice is that of the philosopher John Rawls (1972). Rawls imagines a 'thought experiment' during which a group of individuals are asked to decide on a scheme for a just society, making a collective decision about rights and duties and the distribution of resources in society. In order to achieve this in an impartial way, these individuals are situated in the 'original position' and placed behind a 'veil of ignorance'. This means that, while these individuals have understanding of the natural and the social world, they do not know what position they will occupy in society; they do not know their social status, abilities or disabilities, level of intelligence, occupation or income. Without this knowledge, Rawls assumes that rational individuals will not be guided by subjective self-interest but by rational thought and that they will seek to protect themselves if they find themselves in a disadvantaged situation in society; people will choose principles of justice for the sort of society they would like to inhabit. Rawls suggests that two principles would follow: equal rights for all; and social and economic equality unless inequality is in the interests of all – for example, through the redistribution of wealth.

This situation has been likened to a child being asked to cut a cake fairly when the child does not know which piece they will receive.

Of course, Rawls' theory has been criticised, not least because of his assumption that individuals would behave rationally. However, you can now apply the principles to a 'thought experiment' of your own in order to explore what socially just health policies might look like.

Activity 8.3   *Team working*

Gather together some of your colleagues and attempt Rawls' 'thought experiment'.

How might individuals in the 'original position' plan the provision of healthcare?

What sort of health policies would you design if you did not know what sort of position you would occupy in society? You might be a lawyer with access to private healthcare, or you might be a failed asylum seeker with restricted access to free healthcare. You might be a healthy athlete, or you might suffer from sickle cell disease or diabetes.

There is no answer for this activity. Your discussions will be based on beliefs and opinions, and thus there is no right or wrong answer.

No doubt you aspired to an ideal situation where policies ensure that everyone has equal access to high-quality healthcare. Of course, access to the NHS remains available to everyone, subject to residence conditions, and remains free at the point of delivery. However, there are finite resources available for the NHS, and variations in access to service do exist. Further, as policies are implemented that embed the reforms to the NHS, it is important to be alert to problems and inequalities in service provision. The Chief Executive of the NHS has already stated that the NHS will be on 'high alert'. Ashton (2012, p2) states: *Although there is a commitment to reducing inequalities in health, a whole raft of Coalition Government policies is taking us in the opposite direction.*

There are sound principles and policies to help us ensure the best for our patients: those relating to human rights. In 2008, the Secretary of State for Health stated that *we cannot provide good care without respect for human rights* (DH, 2008d, p2). The DH document *Human rights in healthcare* (DH, 2008d) describes how law relating to human rights is defined at three levels: the international, national and local levels.

International level

Human rights were first defined by the international community in the Universal Declaration of Human Rights in 1948, following the events of the Second World War. Several treaties have followed this Declaration, addressing civil, political, economic, social, cultural and environmental rights. At European level, the Council of Europe adopted the European Convention on Human Rights in 1950. This Convention is the main source of legal human rights protection in the UK, as UK citizens can present human rights cases to the European Court of Human Rights in Strasbourg (DH, 2008d).

National level

In the UK, the 1998 Human Rights Act incorporated the values of fairness, respect, equality, dignity and autonomy into law, and the Act obliges all public services – for example, the NHS – to respect and protect human rights in all their activities. Human rights apply to everyone. The Human Rights Act incorporated most of the rights defined in the European Convention into UK law.

Local level

The NHS has to ensure that all activities are compatible with the provisions of the Human Rights Act: human rights must be at the heart of policy and planning. Fifteen human rights are identified in the Human Rights Act; the rights that apply most readily in healthcare provision are:

- the right to life;
- the right not to be tortured or treated in an inhuman or degrading way;
- the right to respect for private and family life, home and correspondence;
- the right to freedom of thought, conscience and religion;
- the right not to be discriminated against in relation to the enjoyment of any of the rights contained in the European Convention.

It is clear from these rights that an anti-discriminatory stance is adopted, and the Human Rights Act, together with the 2010 Equality Act, provides the framework for nurses to ensure that no patients are discriminated against.

While human rights do apply to everyone, there are certain groups of people who might find it difficult to realise their rights. These 'incomplete' citizens (Rees, 1995) include people with learning disabilities, people with mental health problems, people with dementia, and – as we have already seen in previous chapters – these groups of people are particularly vulnerable and in need of protection.

Implementing policy

We will start by considering quality, which has been the driving force of health and healthcare policy for the New Labour governments (1997–2010) and for the Coalition government. We saw in Chapter 1 how policy is not always implemented as intended. Sometimes there are sound reasons for this, as practitioners adapt policy to suit their patients and locality. Sometimes practitioners fail to implement policy without good reasons; this can have unfavourable consequences.

Nurses are in a strong position to improve the quality of care. However, we have seen that sometimes the quality of care falls below acceptable standards. The inquiry into care provided by Mid Staffordshire NHS Foundation Trust (House of Commons, 2010) found incidents where the standards of basic nursing care were *totally unacceptable*. This inquiry was initiated by the then Secretary of State for Health, Andy Burnham, following concerns about high mortality rates and poor standards of care at Mid Staffordshire NHS Foundation Trust. The inquiry identified systematic failings within the Trust, with low staffing levels and uncaring staff, contributing to a culture that was not conducive to a supportive working environment, and to low morale among staff (House of Commons, 2010). The Trust was also lacking in effective clinical governance. The priorities for the Trust were driven by targets – in particular, targets for waiting times in the accident and emergency department, to the detriment of quality in care. Examples of the problems identified include poor assessment of patients; poor interprofessional working; incomplete nursing records, including nutrition and hydration charts; poor discharge processes. Invariably there are local policies relating to these activities, and it would appear that such policies were not followed. Policies and guidelines often exist to protect patients and nurses, and it is important that they are adhered to.

As long ago as 1999, Scott stressed how clinical governance provides an opportunity for nurses to influence the development of healthcare (Scott, 1999). Clinical governance remains the main vehicle for improving the quality of care. We have already seen that much of the quality agenda set by the Darzi Report *High quality care for all: NHS next stage review final report* (DH, 2008a) remains in place, and the three key elements of safety, patient experience and effectiveness continue to inform policy relating to quality. The Coalition government has adopted an approach that focuses on delivering health outcomes. These are articulated in *The NHS Outcomes Framework 2012/13* (DH, 2011c). The Outcomes Framework allows the Secretary of State for Health to call the NHS Commissioning Board to account in its role of overseeing the commissioning of health services.

The health outcomes are expressed through five domains that encompass safety, patient experience and effectiveness.

1. Preventing people from dying prematurely.
2. Enhancing quality of life for people with long-term conditions.
3. Helping people to recover from episodes of ill health or following injury.
4. Ensuring that people have a positive experience of care.
5. Treating and caring for people in a safe environment and protecting them from avoidable harm.
   (DH, 2011c)

Each of the domains has indicators, improvement areas and supporting NICE quality standards (DH, 2011c). An example of how the Outcomes Framework is translated into practice can be found in *An outcomes strategy for chronic obstructive pulmonary disease (COPD) and asthma in England* (DH, 2011d), which was developed in partnership with a range of stakeholders. The objectives of the strategy are:

• to improve the respiratory health and wellbeing of all communities and minimise inequalities between communities;
• to reduce the number of people who develop COPD by ensuring they are aware of the importance of good lung health and wellbeing, with risk factors understood, avoided or minimised, and by proactively addressing health inequalities;
• to reduce the number of people with COPD who die prematurely through a proactive approach to early identification, diagnosis and intervention, and proactive care and management at all stages of the disease, with a particular focus on the disadvantaged groups and areas with high prevalence;
• to enhance quality of life for people with COPD across all social groups, with a positive, enabling, experience of care and support right through to the end of life;
• to ensure that people with COPD, across all social groups, receive safe and effective care, which minimises progression, enhances recovery and promotes independence;
• to ensure that people with asthma, across all social groups, are free of symptoms because of prompt and accurate diagnosis, shared decision-making regarding treatment, and ongoing support as they self-manage their own condition and to reduce the need for unscheduled healthcare and risk of death;
(DH, 2011d, p10)

It is easy to see how nurses contribute to this strategy through the provision of health promotion, health education and the delivery of nursing care. The following scenario demonstrates this.

Scenario: Frank

Frank is 65 years old. He came to Britain in the 1970s from the Caribbean and has lived in Britain ever since. Frank has suffered mental health problems for the past 30 years, resorted to smoking cigarettes and now has COPD. He has been admitted to hospital with an acute chest infection. In line with the above strategy, the

continued . . .

> *nurses caring for Frank assess his understanding of COPD. They refer Frank to the respiratory nurse to ensure that he is using his inhaler correctly. They involve the physiotherapist, who helps Frank with expectoration, assesses his mobility and teaches him relaxation techniques. The nurses liaise with the doctor treating Frank to ensure accurate reports of his lung function recordings and his response to medications. The nurses ask the occupational therapist to assess Frank's ability to manage at home. They also get in touch with Frank's social worker.*

Nurses also contribute to the knowledge base by carrying out research. The following summary demonstrates how nurses identified a gap in patients' and carers' understanding of COPD and the need for health-promoting activities.

Research summary: promoting the health of people with chronic obstructive pulmonary disease: patients' and carers' views (Caress et al., 2010)

The aim of the research was to gain insights into patients' and carers' understanding of the nature of COPD and the role of health promotion with this population. The researchers conducted interviews with 14 patients and 12 carers. The findings revealed that many participants seemed unaware that their health might benefit from a healthier lifestyle. Patients tended to be stoical and expected to experience symptoms, with little awareness that some interventions might help them. As such, the reality for patients was day-to-day management of symptoms of the disease. Most patients did little to maximise their health beyond participation in pulmonary rehabilitation programmes. However, even when patients did participate in these programmes, few continued the exercises at home. The researchers identified gaps in the patients' and carers' understanding of COPD, the need for ongoing support and the need for effective health promotion.

Governance of quality

In terms of overall governance of quality in the NHS, the Secretary of State for Health remains ultimately accountable to Parliament for the health service in England (DH, 2012f). Commissioners are responsible for commissioning high-quality services to meet the needs of their populations (DH, 2012f). NICE sets national guidelines and standards; the CQC monitors compliance with standards of quality and safety (DH, 2012f). The National Quality Board (NQB) advises the DH on quality across the NHS and at the interface between health and social care services. While the leadership within organisations that provide care remains responsible for the quality of care, healthcare professionals remain the first line of defence in safeguarding quality (DH, 2012f).

In 2010, the Department of Health published *The nursing roadmap for quality* (DH, 2010h). The introduction from the Chief Nursing Officer at the Department of Health states: *Quality is always going to be a key priority for nursing; to deliver quality means nurses working differently – working across pathways, working with other clinical colleagues and working in different environments.* (Beasley, 2010, p1).

However, as well as ensuring quality in nursing care, nurses also need to demonstrate the impact and outcome of nursing care (Beasley, 2010). *The nursing roadmap for quality* uses the seven-step framework to guide improving quality set out in *High quality care for all* (DH, 2008a), and shows how to put these steps into operation using existing mechanisms.

- Bring clarity to quality: this is aided by tools such as quality standards produced by NICE and clinical guidelines.
- Measure quality: quality of care can be measured against tools such as Essence of Care benchmarks and patient feedback.
- Publish quality performance: trusts are required to publish quality accounts to provide information about their performance in relation to quality.
- Recognise and reward quality: improvements in quality can be rewarded through the use of the Commissioning for Quality and Innovation (CQUIN) payment framework. Under this framework a proportion of a service provider's income is conditional on locally agreed quality improvement goals.
- Leadership for quality: leadership for quality is provided by the National Quality Board.
- Safeguard quality: quality is safeguarded by the Care Quality Commission, which is the regulator of all health and adult social care services in England.
- Stay ahead: measures are in place to ensure that innovation continues to keep pace with a dynamic society. These are Academic Health Science Centres and Health Innovation and Education Clusters.

(DH, 2010h, p4)

The following case study demonstrates the power that nurses possess to improve quality of care, and thus make a contribution to the overall policy agenda of quality enhancement.

Case study: nurse-led ward rounds – a valuable contribution to acute stroke care (Catangui and Slark, 2012)

Catangui and Slark (2012) describe the initiation of weekly nurse-led ward rounds in acute stroke care. The ward rounds are led by senior nurses, including a clinical nurse specialist, who assess, examine and evaluate the nursing care provided to patients who have suffered strokes and also stroke outcome measures. During the rounds the team discuss with the nurses caring for the patients' essential nursing care, including the patients' oral care, skin integrity, continence, fluid and nutrition intake, and mood. This process has empowered nurses to make decisions about nursing care within their professional remit. The rounds have contributed to improved communication with the multidisciplinary team, teamwork, patient care and patient experience, as well as early detection of complications.

Influencing policy

West and Scott (2000) argue that nursing activity tends to be viewed as taking place in a 'private' sphere, and stress the need for nurses to have a greater role in the 'public' sphere of policy making. So, how can nurses influence policy? Everyone has the right to put questions to their local Member of Parliament (MP). All MPs hold local surgeries, or you can write to your MP at the House of Commons, asking for a statement on their position on a particular health issue, or providing information on your position. Fyffe (2009) suggests measures to enhance the nurse's role in relation to policy, including education, research and engaging in the media. However, as stated by the ICN (2011, p43):

> *National nursing associations provide a means by which nurses' interests can be articulated and provide a first point of contact with key stakeholders in government and civil society, and are key to the development of an effective contribution to policy debates on both how the health system is oriented, structured and managed, but also on broader policy issues which address the social determinants of health.*

We have already seen in Chapter 1 how the RCN lobbied Parliament during the passage of the Health and Social Care Act and how it joined forces with other professional organisations in order to maximise impact and show a united front. It is important, therefore, to belong to, and support, a professional organisation – that is, the RCN. With the changing landscape of health policy there are plenty of opportunities for organisations to get involved (Fyffe, 2009), and membership of a professional organisation ensures contact with active campaigning networks. In order to influence policy, nurses might also develop social networks that involve researchers and policy makers (West and Scott, 2000).

Evidence-based policy

Maben and Griffiths (2008) argue that in order to ensure high-quality care the nursing profession needs to *recast the role of the nurse as a practitioner, partner and leader,* within the context of a new professionalism centred round caring and the patient experience. Antrobus (2003) describes how nursing leaders can influence policy by taking account of evidence, experiences of caring for patients and service user perspectives. Antrobus draws a useful analogy with the growth of research capacity in nursing: just as every nurse needs to be research aware in order to translate research findings into practice, so every nurse needs to be policy aware in order to translate policy into practice (Antrobus, 2003).

We have already seen that there is a requirement for policy to be evidence-based, and Glasby (2006) calls for policy to be informed by the *practice wisdom of health and social care practitioners,* together with feedback from service users, alongside the more traditional and scientific forms of evidence. Several writers have stressed the importance of research in influencing policy (West and Scott, 2000; Daly et al., 2004). However, little is known about the influence of nursing research on health policy (Bunn and Kendall, 2011). Bunn and Kendall explored whether nursing research does have an impact on policy.

Research summary: 'Does nursing research impact on policy? A case study of health visiting research and UK health policy' (Bunn and Kendall, 2011)

The study aimed to explore the impact of nursing research on the development of health-care policy. The researchers used documentary and literature reviews, citation analysis and interviews with researchers to explore the impact of health-visiting research on UK health policy. The research found that there was evidence of health-visiting research influencing healthcare policy but that it was limited. Many of the studies cited in policy documents were qualitative, and there was a lack of evaluative research, in particular, randomised controlled trials – the gold standard of scientific research.

The rational approach to policy making is appealing. According to this approach, policy makers identify a problem, search for relevant research, decide on what works and then implement the evidence (Glasby, 2011). However, policy is not always based on evidence and, as we have seen, is often the outcome of demands from different stakeholders (Elliott and Popay, 2000; Daly et al., 2004; Bunn and Kendall, 2011; Glasby, 2011). Elliott and Popay's (2000) study of research utilisation in NHS policy making in one NHS region in England revealed a tendency for research to have an indirect influence on policy by shaping policy debate and dialogue between service providers and users.

The opportunities are now available to conduct research as the Coalition government's reforms are implemented in order to be able to feed back information on the effects of the reforms on patient care. One way forward might be through the use of patient stories. Nurses are accustomed to using patient stories to shape practice and to improve the quality of care. With the attention that is being paid to service user and public involvement in health policy formulation, maybe now is the time to use such stories to inform policy.

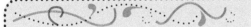

Chapter summary

Not all nurses can become movers and shakers in health policy terms, but nurses do need to be aware of policy and knowledgeable about policy that affects their field of practice. This chapter has provided examples of ways of developing policy awareness and knowledge. Most nurses are implementing policy in their daily work, but may not always be aware of it. Suggestions have been made concerning how to influence policy; this is most effective if carried out through professional organisations.

Activities: Brief outline answers

Activity 8.1: Critical thinking (page 138)

You might have decided that policy awareness is important in order to be able to discuss current policy with patients if they ask questions. After all, current policy is widely available to the public through the television, newspapers and the internet. You might also have highlighted the need to be aware of the most recent guidelines relating to your area of practice, or the need to be aware in order to be able to influence policy. There are, of course, also the general policy requirements to improve the quality of care and patient safety.

Further reading

Bunn, F and Kendall, S (2011) Does nursing research impact on policy? A case study of health visiting research and UK health policy. *Journal of Research in Nursing*, 16(2): 169–91.

This article has an interesting discussion of the impact of research on policy.

Ellis, P (2010) *Evidence-based practice in nursing*. Exeter: Learning Matters.

This book equips nurses with the knowledge and skills required to appraise and apply evidence in their practice.

Fyffe, T (2009) Nursing shaping and influencing health and social care policy. *Journal of Nursing Management*, 17: 698–706.

This article addresses the developing role of the nurse in relation to health policy and reports on lessons learnt from the USA.

Useful website

www.equalityhumanrights.com

The website of the Equality and Human Rights Commission gives more information on human rights.

Glossary

active failures   errors that are immediately apparent. They include slips, lapses, mistakes and violations of procedures, guidelines and policies.

adverse event   an event that leads to serious patient harm or death.

asylum seeker   someone who has applied for refugee status in a host country and is awaiting a decision on the application. The distinction between a 'refugee' and an 'asylum seeker' is important because the status of asylum seeker attracts fewer rights and benefits than that of a refugee.

Big Society   concerns community involvement to improve people's lives. It entails a transfer of power from central government to local communities.

care pathways   structured integrated plans for organising patient care processes and outcomes in particular settings.

Care Quality Commission (CQC)   regulatory body alongside Monitor (see below) to ensure that services meet safety and quality standards.

care trusts   established to focus on integrated services for particular groups – for example, older people, people with mental health problems or people with learning difficulties. Care trusts represent a single organisation within the NHS but deliver both health and social care services.

Clinical Commissioning Groups (CCGs)   the groups that take over the responsibilities of Primary Care Trusts (PCTs) from April 2013. They will commission and buy health and care services for their patients. As well as GPs, CCGs will include nurses, hospital doctors and members of the public.

commissioner–provider split   replaced the *purchaser–provider split* (see below). GP fund-holding proved to be divisive, but the Labour government (1997) recognised the benefits of the principles of a purchaser-provider split. This government discontinued the practice of GP fund-holding and competition, and replaced it with local commissioning bodies (Primary Care Trusts) with an emphasis on planning and collaboration.

community alarm   an alarm, sometimes called a personal alarm, that an individual wears around their neck and that is linked, via the telephone, to a local social care office. If the individual needs assistance – for example, if they have fallen over – they can press the alarm, and this alerts the social care services team.

democratic deficit   refers to the early years when the NHS lacked directly elected representatives – senior managerial staff tended to be appointed by the Secretary of State for Health. The situation was often contrasted with local government, which has locally elected councillors. This perceived deficit led to initiatives to increase local decision-making, and increased lay representation on NHS committees.

democratic socialism   see social democracy.

fund-holding general practitioners   introduced in the 1990s as part of the *internal market* for healthcare (see below). Fund-holding GPs were given their own budgets in order to purchase care for their patients from a range of providers. Not all GP practices chose to become fund-holders. The scheme proved to have the potential to contribute to inequalities, as fund-holding GPs had more power in terms of purchasing services for their patients.

general management   an approach that was introduced into the NHS in the 1980s against the desire to restrain public spending and adopt a more managerial approach. General managers were employed at all levels of the NHS to improve leadership, responsibility and accountability.

Health Action Zones (HAZs)   zones established in 1998 in order to improve the health of people in areas of deprivation and poor health. Their aim was to reduce inequalities in health through inter-agency collaboration and responding to the needs of local populations.

Health Improvement Programmes (HImPs)   programmes established in the late 1990s that focused on promoting health as well as improving healthcare. Local health authorities were required to engage with local authorities to formulate these plans.

Healthwatch England   the national consumer champion for health and social care in England. It is part of a HealthWatch network. There is a local HealthWatch organisation in every local authority area, whose role is to seek the views of local communities on health and social care services. These views are then fed back to HealthWatch England which identifies key issues and trends and ensures that the voices of local people are used to inform policy.

iatrogenic illness   illness that is caused by medicine – for example, illness that arises from side effects of treatments.

Independent Sector Treatment Centres (ISTCs)   developed as part of the collaboration between the NHS and the independent sector. These centres are often located on the sites of NHS hospitals and perform diagnostic functions and elective surgery. These centres undertake work on behalf of the NHS and they can be run by overseas companies.

internal market   introduced by Mrs. Thatcher in the 1990s. The internal market increased competition in the NHS and allowed hospitals (NHS and private sector) to compete with each other for contracts with GPs.

latent conditions   in the context of patient safety, the underlying conditions that lie dormant in a system and are not immediately apparent. They are conditions that, when combined with other factors, allow active failures to occur.

means testing   the process that is used to determine if an individual has the 'means', for example, money or resources, to meet their own needs, or if they are eligible for government help, in terms of paying a reduced price or receiving a government subsidy. Stigma is sometimes attached to means-testing.

Monitor   a body with a regulatory role alongside the CQC (see above). Its role is to promote efficiency and ensure that competition within the NHS works in patients' interests. Monitor also supports continuity of services and has the power to set prices.

National Health Service Commissioning Board (NHS Commissioning Board)   a body that oversees the commissioning activities of Clinical Commissioning Groups. The Board allocates resources to the CCGs and commissions certain services itself, for example, primary care.

National Health Service Outcomes Framework   a framework that defines national outcomes that the NHS should aim to improve as part of the quality enhancement agenda. It provides a national overview of how the NHS is performing and can be used by the Secretary of State for Health to call the NHS Commissioning Board to account.

National Health Service Trusts   first created in the 1990s out of existing NHS services, typically hospitals. When they became trusts, hospitals were no longer under the direct management of health authorities. They remained part of the NHS, but had greater freedom to manage their services. Trust status is now universal.

National Institute for Health and Clinical Excellence (NICE)   an independent organisation that was established in 1999. Its remit includes reducing variations in access to treatments on the basis of where people live. NICE produces national evidence-based guidelines for the treatment of different conditions, and its role is now extended to social care.

National Service Frameworks (NSFs)   frameworks that define standards of care and care pathways for specific conditions and patient groups, and include evidence-based guidance on treatment and services.

near miss   a patient safety incident that has been prevented. The problem has been identified and rectified.

neo-liberalism   refers to the importance of markets, private property, the freedom of individuals and minimal government. The policies of the Conservative party led by Mrs Thatcher were influenced by neo-liberalism, for example, through the introduction of the internal market (see above).

Ombudsman   The Parliamentary and Health Service Ombudsman service is an independent service that considers complaints against government departments, public bodies in the UK and the NHS in England, in relation to unfair or poor provision of services.

policy community   refers to the set of 'actors', from the public and private spheres, who influence policy design and implementation.

Private Finance Initiatives (PFIs)   part of the reforms that aimed to increase the role of the private sector in financing healthcare. Under PFIs, the private sector is used to raise funds for capital development in the NHS (rather than using public funds), typically to build a new hospital.

purchaser–provider split   a division between purchasers and providers of healthcare services, introduced as part of the *internal market*. Patient services were purchased from providers by fundholding GPs or by District Health Authorities (on behalf of non-fundholding GPs). Purchasers could draw up contracts with their preferred providers.

refugee   According to the United Nations Convention Relating to the Status of Refugees (1951), and its 1967 Protocol, a refugee is a person who: *Owing to a well-founded fear of being persecuted for reasons of race, religion, nationality, membership of a particular social group or political opinion, is outside the country of his nationality and is unable, or owing to such fear, is unwilling to avail himself of the protection of that country* . . .. In practical terms, a refugee is a person who has been granted refugee status in a host country, within the terms of the above Convention.

social capital   refers to social integration (as opposed to isolation) and the good that people acquire from having supportive social relations and social networks.

social democracy   a political ideology that favours state involvement in social and economic life, for example, through a welfare state. Social democrats favour equality and solidarity.

social enterprises   organisations that are run like business but with social intentions. Any profit made by social enterprises is put back into the business or the community it serves. Social enterprises are able to use innovative ways to meet local needs.

telecare   a range of person-centred remote-care technologies that are available for people with long-term conditions. These technologies aim to help people to remain independent in their own homes. They include personal alarms, health monitoring devices and sensors that can alert carers to changes taking place within the home, for example, if a person with dementia leaves the house.

third sector   the range of organisations that do not fall within either the public or the private sector. It includes voluntary and community organisations.

third way   somewhere between social democracy and neo-liberalism, described in the politics of Tony Blair as somewhere between the traditional social democracy of the post-war Labour government and the New Right approach of the Conservative party of Mrs Thatcher. For example, the New Labour government was committed to equality and the welfare state, but aimed to reduce dependency on the state, expressed through the slogan *no rights without responsibilities*.

References

Acheson, D (1998) *Independent inquiry into inequalities in health*. London: Stationery Office.

Age Concern (2006) *Hungry to be heard*. London: Age Concern.

Age Concern (2010) *Still hungry to be heard*. London: Age Concern.

Ager, A (1999) Perspectives on the refugee experience, in Ager, A (ed.) *Refugees: perspectives on the experience of forced migration*. London: Cassell.

Alexis, O (2005) Managing change: cultural diversity in the NHS workforce. *Nursing Management*, 11(10): 28–30.

Antrobus, S (2003) What is political leadership? *Nursing Standard*, 17(43): 40–44.

Arnstein, SR (1969) A ladder of citizen participation. *Journal of the American Planning Association*, 35(4): 216–24.

Ashton, JR (2012) Defending democracy and the National Health Service. *The Lancet*, Early Online Publication, 24 February. doi:10.1016/S0140–6736(12)60287–6.

Baggott, R (2000) *Public health: policy and politics*. Basingstoke: Macmillan Press.

Baggott, R (2004) *Health and health care in Britain* (3rd edn). Basingstoke: Palgrave Macmillan.

Baggott, R (2007) *Understanding health policy*. Bristol: Policy Press.

Balarajan, R (1996) Ethnicity and variations in mortality from coronary heart disease. *Health Trends*, 28(2): 45–51.

Balarajan, R and Soni Raleigh, V (1993) *Ethnicity and health: a guide for the NHS*. London: Department of Health.

Barbalet, JM (1988) *Citizenship*. Milton Keynes: Open University Press.

Barham, L and Devlin, N (2011) Patient-reported outcome measures: implications for nursing. *Nursing Standard*, 25(18): 42–45.

Barnes, M (1999) Users as citizens: Collective action and the local governance of welfare. *Social Policy and Administration*, 33(1): 73–90.

Barnes, M and Walker, A (1996) Consumerism versus empowerment: a principled approach to the involvement of older service users. *Policy and Politics*, 24(4): 375–93.

Barrett, G, Sellman, D and Thomas, J (2005) Introduction, in Barrett, G., Sellman, D and Thomas, J (eds) *Interprofessional working in health and social care: professional perspectives*. Basingstoke: Palgrave Macmillan.

Baxter, SK and Brumfitt, SM (2008) Professional differences in interprofessional working. *Journal of Interprofessional Care*, 22(3): 239–51.

BBC News (2012) NHS bill: GPs offer to help with health changes. 13 March. Available at: www.bbc.co.uk/news/health-17348616 (accessed 13 March).

Beasley, C (2010) Introduction, in Department of Health (2010) *The nursing roadmap for quality: a signposting map for nursing*. London: Department of Health.

Beaumont, K, Luettel, D and Thomson, R (2008) Deterioration in hospital patients: early signs and appropriate actions. *Nursing Standard*, 23(1): 43–8.

Beresford, P (2005) Service user: regressive or liberatory terminology? *Disability & Society*, 20(4): 469–77.

Beresford, P and Croft, S (1993) *Citizen involvement: a practical guide for change*. London: Macmillan.

Bergen, A and While, A (2005) 'Implementation deficit' and 'street-level bureaucracy': policy, practice and change in the development of community nursing issues. *Health and Social Care in the Community*, 13(1): 1–10.

Bhopal, R, Unwin, N, White, M, Yallop, J, Walker, L, Alberti, KGMM, Harland, J, Patel, S, Ahmad, N, Turner, C, Watson, B, Kaur, D, Kulkarni, A, Laker, M and Tavridou, A (1999) Heterogeneity of coronary heart disease risk factors in Indian, Pakistani, Bangladeshi, and European origin populations: cross sectional study. *British Medical Journal*, 319: 215–20.

Bird, D (2005) Patient safety: improving incident reporting. *Nursing Standard*, 20(14–16): 43–6.

Bird, D and Dennis, S (2005) Integrating risk management into working practice. *Nursing Standard*, 20(13): 52–4.

Blakemore, K (2003) *Social policy: an introduction.* Buckingham: Open University Press.

Boseley, S (2010) Tories prescribe a dose of data as panacea for choice in NHS. *The Guardian*, 13 July: 6–7.

Boseley, S (2012) Work stress can raise risk of heart attack by 23%, study finds. *The Guardian*, 14 September.

Bosma, H, Marmot, MG, Hemingway, H, Nicholson, AC, Brunner, E and Stansfield, SA (1997) Low job control and risk of coronary heart disease in Whitehall II (prospective cohort) study. *British Medical Journal*, 314: 558–65.

Bowcott, O (2009) Jayne Zito: why it's time to end campaign. *The Observer*, 17 May.

Boyle, G (2010) Social policy for people with dementia in England: promoting human rights? *Health and Social Care in the Community*, 18(5): 511–19.

Bradbury-Jones, C (2009) Globalisation and its implications for health care and nursing practice. *Nursing Standard*, 23(25): 43–7.

Braine, ME (2006) Clinical governance: applying theory to practice. *Nursing Standard*, 20(20): 56–65.

Braithwaite, J, Runciman, WB and Merry, AF (2009) Towards safer, better healthcare: harnessing the natural properties of complex sociotechnical systems. *Quality and Safety in Health Care*, 18: 37–41.

Brodie, E, Hughes, T, Jochum, V, Miller, S, Ockenden, N and Warburton, D (2011) *Pathways through participation: what creates and sustains active citizenship?* London: NCVO, IVR and Involve.

Brown, M, MacArthur, J, McKechanie, A, Hayes, M and Fletcher, J (2010) Equality and access to general health care for people with learning disabilities: reality or rhetoric? *Journal of Research in Nursing*, 15(4): 351–61.

Brown, PR (2008) Trusting in the new NHS: instrumental *versus* communicative action. *Sociology of Health & Illness*, 30(3): 349–63.

Brownlie, J and Howson, A (2008) Introduction, in Brownlie, J, Greene, A and Howson, A (eds) *Researching trust and health.* Abingdon: Routledge.

Bryant, R (2011) Influencing and persuading: the need to increase government access to nursing policy advice. *International Nursing Review*, 58(2): 148.

Bunn, F and Kendall, S (2011) Does nursing research impact on policy? A case study of health visiting research and UK health policy. *Journal of Research in Nursing*, 16(2): 169–91.

Burchardt, T and Craig, G (2008) Introduction, in Craig, G, Burchardt, T and Gordon, D (eds) *Social justice and public policy: seeking fairness in diverse societies.* Bristol: The Policy Press.

Buse, K, Mays, N and Walt, G (2005) *Making health policy.* Maidenhead: Open University Press.

Cabinet Office (2010) *The Coalition: our programme for government.* London: Her Majesty's Government.

Calnan, M and Rowe, R (2008) *Trust matters in health care.* Maidenhead: Open University Press.

Calnan, MW and Sanford, E (2004) Public trust in health care: the system or the doctor? *Quality and Safety in Health Care*, 13: 92–7.

Cambridge, J (2008) Managing risk and improving patient safety in clinical practice: reducing medication errors. Healthcare Events, Manchester Conference Centre, Manchester, 20 March 2008. *Diversity in Health and Social Care*, 5(2): 166–7.

Cameron, D and Clegg, N (2010) Foreword, in Cabinet Office *The Coalition: our programme for government.* London: Her Majesty's Government.

Campbell, D (2010) Private companies see potential to expand their role. *The Guardian*, 13 July: 6–7.

Campbell, D (2011) Some elderly NHS patients left with little to eat or drink, watchdog finds. *The Guardian*, 26 May, p10.

Campbell, S. (2007) The need for a global response to antimicrobial resistance. *Nursing Standard*, 21(44): 35–40.

Car, J, Black, A, Anandan, C, Cresswell, K, Pagliari, C, McKinstry, B, Procter, R, Majeed, A and Sheikh, A (2008) *The impact of eHealth on the quality and safety of healthcare.* London: Imperial College.

Carers UK (2009) *Facts about carers.* London: Carers UK.

Carers UK (2011) *Valuing carers 2011. Calculating the value of carers' support.* London: Carers UK.

Caress, A, Luker, K and Chalmers, K (2010) Promoting the health of people with chronic obstructive pulmonary disease: patients' and carers' views. *Journal of Clinical Nursing*, 19: 564–73.

Carter, P, Meldrum, H, Jennings, K, Reay, K, Warwick, C and Gray, P (2011) Letter. *The Times*, 17 January.

Carvel, J (2008) Nurses to be rated on how compassionate and smiley they are. *The Guardian*, 18 June.

Carvel, J (2009) Man with Down's syndrome dies after starving for 26 days in hospital. *The Guardian*, 24 March.

Catangui, EJ and Slark, J (2012) Nurse-led ward rounds: a valuable contribution to acute stroke care. *British Journal of Nursing*, 21(13): 801–5.

Cheater, FM (2010) Improving primary and community health services through nurse-led social enterprise. *Quality in Primary Care*, 18: 5–7.

Coid, JW (1994) The Christopher Clunis enquiry. *Psychiatric Bulletin*, 18: 449–52.

Collins, F and McCray, J (2012) Partnership working in services for children: use of the common assessment framework. *Journal of Interprofessional Care*. 26: 134–40.

Colyer, HM (2004) The construction and development of health professions: where will it end? *Journal of Advanced Nursing*, 48(4): 406–12.

Commission on Dignity in Care (2012) *Delivering dignity: securing dignity in care for older people in hospitals and care homes*. Available at: www.nhsconfed.org/Publications/Documents/Delivering_Dignity_final_report 150612.pdf.

Commission on Social Justice (1994) *Social justice: strategies for national renewal*. London: Vintage.

Cooper, L, Coote, A, Davies, A and Jackson, C (1995) *Voices off: tackling the democratic deficit in health*. London: IPPR.

Coulter, A and Collins, A (2011) *Making shared decision-making a reality: no decision about me, without me*. London: The King's Fund. Available at: www.kingsfund.org.uk/publications/nhs_decisionmaking.html.

Council of Europe (2010) *White Paper on intercultural dialogue: living together as equals in dignity*. Strasbourg: Council of Europe. Available at: www.coe.int/t/dg4/intercultural/publication_whitepaper_id_en.asp.

Council of the European Union (2009) Council Recommendation of 9 June 2009 on patient safety, including the prevention and control of healthcare associated infections. (2009/C151/01). *Official Journal of the European Union*, 3.7.2009. Luxembourg.

Cowan, DT and Norman, I (2006) Cultural competence in nursing: new meanings. *Journal of Transcultural Nursing*, 17(1): 82–8.

CQC (Care Quality Commission) (2011a) *Dignity and nutrition inspection programme. National overview*. London: Care Quality Commission.

CQC (2011b) *Internal management review of the regulation of Winterbourne View*. London: Care Quality Commission.

CSDH (Commission on Social Determinants of Health) (2008) *Closing the gap in a generation: health equity through action on the social determinants of health*. Geneva: World Health Organisation. Available at: www.who.int/social_determinants/final_report/en/index.html.

Currie, L. (2000) National service frameworks: what are they? *Nursing Standard*, 14(41): 43–5.

Dalrymple, J and Burke, B (1995) *Anti-oppressive practice: social care and the law*. Milton Keynes: Open University Press.

Daly, J, Thompson, DR, Chang, E and Hancock, K (2004) The context of nursing and health care research, in Crookes, PA and Davies, S (eds) *Research into practice* (2nd edn). Edinburgh: Baillière Tindall.

Daly, M (2002) Care as a good for social policy. *Journal of Social Policy*, 31(2): 251–70.

Davidson, J, Baxter, K, Glendinning, C, Jones, K, Forder, J, Caiels, J, Welch, E, Windle, K, Dolan, P and King, D (2012) *Personal health budgets: experiences and outcomes for budget holders at nine months. Fifth Interim Report*. London: Department of Health.

Department for Constitutional Affairs (2007) *Mental Capacity Act 2005. Code of Practice*. London: The Stationery Office. Available at: www.justice.gov.uk./protecting-the-vulnerable/mental-capacity-act.

Department for Education (2010) *Working together to safeguard children: a guide to inter-agency working to safeguard and promote the welfare of children*. London: Department for Education.

Department for Education and Skills (2003) *Every child matters*. London: HMSO.

DH (Department of Health) (1989) *Caring for people: community care in the next decade and beyond*. London: Department of Health.

DH (1997) *The new NHS: modern, dependable.* Norwich: The Stationery Office.

DH (1998a) *A first class service: quality in the new NHS.* London: Department of Health.

DH (1998b) *Our healthier nation: a contract for health.* London: Department of Health.

DH (1999) *Caring about carers: a national strategy for carers.* London: Department of Health.

DH (2000a) *NHS Plan: a plan for investment; a plan for reform.* London: Department of Health.

DH (2000b) *An organisation with a memory: report of an expert group on learning from adverse events in the NHS chaired by the Chief Medical Officer.* London: The Stationery Office.

DH (2000c) *The NHS cancer plan: a plan for investment, a plan for reform.* London: Department of Health.

DH (2001a) *National Service Framework for older people.* London: Department of Health.

DH (2001b) *Shifting the balance of power.* London: Department of Health.

DH (2001c) *Involving patients and the public in healthcare: a discussion document.* London: Department of Health.

DH (2001d) *The expert patient: a new approach to chronic disease management for the 21st century.* London: Department of Health.

DH (2003) *The Victoria Climbié Inquiry: report of an inquiry by Lord Laming.* Cm 5730. London: Department of Health.

DH (2006a) *Our health, our care, our say: a new direction for community services.* Norwich: The Stationery Office.

DH (2006b) *Safety first: a report for patients, clinicians and healthcare managers.* London: The Stationery Office.

DH (2007) *National stroke strategy.* London: Department of Health.

DH (2008a) *High quality care for all: NHS next stage review final report.* Norwich: The Stationery Office.

DH (2008b) *End of life care strategy: promoting high quality care for all adults at the end of life.* London: Department of Health.

DH (2008c) *Guidance on the routine collection of Patient Reported Outcome Measures (PROMs).* London: Department of Health.

DH (2008d) *Human rights in healthcare: a framework for local action* (2nd edn). London: Department of Health.

DH (2009a) *Living well with dementia: a National Dementia Strategy.* London: Department of Health.

DH (2009b) *Valuing people now: a new 4 year strategy for people with learning disabilities.* London: Department of Health.

DH (2010a) *Equity and excellence: liberating the NHS.* Norwich: The Stationery Office.

DH (2010b) *Ready to go? Planning the discharge and transfer of patients from hospital and intermediate care.* London: Department of Health.

DH (2010c) *Press releases. Health Secretary sets out ambition for a culture of patient safety in the NHS.* London: Department of Health. Available at: www.dh.gov.uk/en/MediaCentre/Pressreleases/DH_116634.

DH (2010d) *Essence of Care 2010: benchmarks for respect and dignity.* Norwich: The Stationery Office.

DH (2010e) *How to use Essence of Care 2010.* Norwich: The Stationery Office.

DH (2010f) *Healthy lives, health people: our strategy for public health in England.* London: The Stationery Office.

DH (2010g) *Our health and wellbeing today.* London: Department of Health.

DH (2010h) *The nursing roadmap for quality.* London: Department of Health.

DH (2011a) *Safeguarding adults: the role of health service practitioners.* London: Department of Health.

DH (2011b) *Health lives, healthy people: a call to action on obesity in England.* London: Department of Health.

DH (2011c) *The NHS Outcomes Framework 2012/13.* London: Department of Health.

DH (2011d) *An outcomes strategy for chronic obstructive pulmonary disease (COPD) and asthma in England.* London: Department of Health.

DH (2012a) *Delivering the NHS Safety Thermometer CQUIN 2012/13: a preliminary guide to measuring 'harm free' care.* London: Department of Health.

DH (2012b) *The NHS Constitution.* London: Department of Health.

DH (2012c) *Prime Minister's challenge on dementia: delivering major improvements in dementia care and research by 2015.* London: Department of Health.

DH (2012d) *Understanding personal health budgets.* London: Department of Health.

DH (2012e) *The Family Nurse Partnership Programme. Information Leaflet.* Available at: www.dh.gov.uk/health/2012/07/family-nurse-partnership-programme-information-leaflet/.

DH (2012f) *Quality in the new health system: maintaining and improving quality from April 2012. A draft report from the National Quality Board.* London: Department of Health.

DHSSPS (Department of Health, Social Services and Public Safety) (2005) *Equal lives: review of policy and services for people with a learning disability in Northern Ireland.* Available at: www.dhsspsni.gov.uk/learning-disability-report.

Dix, G, Phillips, J and Braide, M (2012) Engaging staff with intentional rounding. *Nursing Times*, 108(3): 14–16.

Donaldson, L (2003) Expert patients usher in a new era of opportunity for the NHS. *British Medical Journal*, 326: 1279.

Duncan, B (2002) Health policy in the European Union: how it's made and how to influence it. *British Medical Journal*, 324(7344): 1027–30.

Ellershaw, JE and Wilkinson, S (2011) *Care of the dying: a pathway to excellence* (2nd edn). Oxford: Oxford University Press.

Elliott, H and Popay, J (2000) How are policy makers using evidence? Models of research utilisation and local NHS policy making. *Journal of Epidemiology and Community Health*, 54(6): 461–8.

Entwistle, VA and Quick, O (2006) Trust in the context of patient safety problems. *Journal of Health Organisation and Management*, 20(5): 397–416.

European Commission (2005) *Luxembourg Declaration on patient safety*. European Commission. Available at: http://ec.europa.eu/health/ph_overview/Documents/ev_20050405_rd01_en.pdf.

Fenwick, A (2010) Clinical Ethics Committee Case II: is the insertion of a percutaneous endoscopic gastrostomy in our patient's best interests? *Clinical Ethics*, 5: 118–21.

Fink, J (2004) Questions of care, in Fink, J (ed.) *Care. personal lives and social policy*. Bristol: The Policy Press in association with the Open University.

Fortier, JP (2008) Cultural and linguistic competence: a global issue. *Diversity in Health and Social Care*, 5(2): 87–8.

Frowe, I (2005) Professional trust. *British Journal of Educational Studies*, 53(1): 34–53.

Fyffe, T (2009) Nursing shaping and influencing health and social care policy. *Journal of Nursing Management*, 17: 698–706.

Gaskell, S and Nightingale, S (2010) Supporting people with learning disabilities in acute care. *Nursing Standard*, 24(18): 42–8.

Giddens, A (1998) *The third way: the renewal of social democracy*. Oxford: Polity Press.

Gijón-Sánchez, M, Pinzón-Pulido, S, Kolehmainen-Aitken, R, Weekers, J, Aucuña, DL, Benedict, R and Peiro, M (2010) Better health for all in Europe: developing a migrant sensitive health workforce. *Eurohealth*, 16(1): 17.

Gillen, S (2010) Community nurses ill-informed over transfer to social enterprises. *Nursing Standard*. 25(2): 9.

Gilson, L (2003) Trust and the development of health care as a social institution. *Social Science & Medicine*, 56: 1453–68.

Glasby, J (2006) Who knows best? Evidence-based practice and the service user contribution. *Critical Social Policy*, 26(1): 268–84.

Glasby, J (2007) *Understanding health and social care*. Bristol: The Policy Press.

Glasby, J (2011) *Evidence, policy and practice: critical perspectives in health and social care*. Bristol: The Policy Press.

Glasby, J and Dickinson, H (2008) *Partnership working in health and social care*. Bristol: The Policy Press.

Glasby, J, Martin, G and Regen, E (2008) Older people and the relationship between hospital services and intermediate care: results from a national evaluation. *Journal of Interprofessional Care*, 22(6): 639–49.

Goddard, AF (2011) The professional qualifications directive Green Paper: a UK physicians' perspective. *Eurohealth*, 17(4): 7–10.

Goddard, M and Smith, P (2001) Equity of access to health care services: theory and evidence from the UK. *Social Science & Medicine*, 53: 1149–62.

Graham, H and Kelly, MP (2004) *Briefing paper. Health inequalities: concepts, frameworks and policy*. London: Health Development Agency.

Green, J and Thorogood, N (1998) *Analysing health policy: a sociological approach*. London: Longman.

Greenwell, J (1996) Sociology of the NHS: when does the community decide? In Perry, A (ed.) *Sociology: insights in health care*. London: Arnold.

Ham, C and Smith, J (2010) *Removing the policy barriers to integrated care in England*. London: The Nuffield Trust.

Ham, C and Curry, N (2011) *Integrated care. What is it? Does it work? What does it mean for the NHS?* London: The King's Fund.

Harris, D (2012) Care pathway used to 'cut costs' claim doctors. *The Independent*, 9 July.

Harris, J (2002) Caring for citizenship. *British Journal of Social Work*, 32: 267–81.

Harrison, S and Mort, M (1998) Which champions? Which people? Public and user involvement in healthcare as a technology of legitimation. *Social Policy and Administration*, 32(1): 60–70.

HEA (Health Education Authority) (1994) *Black and minority ethnic groups in England: health and lifestyles*. London: HEA.

Healthcare Commission (2009) *Safely does it: implementing safer care for patients*. London: Healthcare Commission.

Hearnden, M (2008) Coping with differences in culture and communication in health care. *Nursing Standard*, 23(11): 49–57.

Help the Hospices (2012) *Towards excellence in hospice care: widening access through nurse leadership. Guidance and resources for professionals*. London: Help the Hospices.

Her Majesty's Government (2012a) *Caring for our future: reforming care and support. Cm 8378*. Norwich: The Stationery Office.

Her Majesty's Government (2012b) *No health without mental health: implementation framework*. London: Her Majesty's Government.

Hervey, T (2010) The impacts of European Union law on the health care sector. *Eurohealth*, 16(4): 5–7.

Hingley-Jones, H and Allain, L (2008) Integrating services for disabled children and their families in two English local authorities. *Journal of Interprofessional Care*, 22(5): 534–44.

Hinsliff, G (2008a) GPs defeat 'health tourist' clampdown. *The Observer*, 12 October: 2.

Hinsliff, G (2008b) GPs attack ban on asylum seekers. *The Observer*, 3 August: 5.

Hirschman, AO (1970) *Exit, voice and loyalty: responses to decline in firms, organisations, and states*. London: Harvard University Press.

Hopkins, A (2012) From a service to a business: the development of a social enterprise. *Primary Health Care*, 22(6): 24–6.

House of Commons (2010) *Independent Inquiry into care provided by Mid Staffordshire NHS Foundation Trust January 2005–March 2009*. Chaired by Robert Francis QC. London: The Stationery Office. Available at: www.midstaffsinquiry.com.

House of Commons Health Committee (2011) *Annual accountability hearing with the Nursing and Midwifery Council. Seventh Report of Session 2010–12*. London: The Stationery Office.

HPA (Health Protection Agency) (2011) *Migrant health: infectious diseases in non-UK born populations in the UK. An update to the baseline report – 2011*. London: Health Protection Agency.

Hudson, B (1998) Take your partners. *Health Service Journal*, 108(5590): 30–1.

Hudson, B (2002) Interprofessionality in health and social care: the Achilles' heel of partnership? *Journal of Interprofessional Care*, 16(1): 7–17.

Hudson, B and Henwood, M (2002) The NHS and social care: the final countdown? *Policy & Politics*, 30(2): 153–66.

Hunter, DJ (2003) *Public health policy*. Oxford: Polity Press.

Hupe, P and Hill, M (2007) Street-level bureaucracy and public accountability. *Public Administration*, 85(2): 279–99.

Hynes, T (2003) *The issue of 'trust' or 'mistrust' in research with refugees: choices, caveats and considerations for researchers. New issues in refugee research*. Working Paper No. 98. Geneva: UNHCR.

ICN (International Council of Nurses) (2011) *Closing the gap: increasing access and equity*. Geneva: ICN. Available at: www.icn.ch/publications/2011-closing-the-gap-increasing-access-and-equity/.

Insight Research Group (2012) *The Austerity Britain Report: the impact of the recession on the UK's health, according to GPs*. Available at: www.insightrg.com/downloads/austerity-britain-key-findings-august-2012.pdf.

Irwin, R. (2010) EU law and health: an introduction. *Eurohealth*, 16(4): 1–2.

Jeffreys, B and Triggle, B (2012) NHS 'on high alert during change'. 27 September. Available at: www.bbc.co.uk/news/health-19729970 (accessed 28 September 2012).

Johns, JL (1996) A concept analysis of trust. *Journal of Advanced Nursing*, 24: 76–83.

Johnson, P, Wistow, G, Schulz, R and Hardy, B (2003) Interagency and interprofessional collaboration in community care: the interdependence of structures and values. *Journal of Interprofessional Care*, 17(1): 69–83.

Johnstone, M and Kanitsaki, O (2006) Culture, language, and patient safety: making the link. *International Journal for Quality in Health Care*, 18(5): 383–8.

Jones, K (2000) *The making of social policy in Britain* (3rd edn). London: The Athlone Press.

Jones, K, Brown, J and Bradshaw, J (1983) *Issues in social policy*. London: Routledge and Kegan Paul.

Jones, SP, Auton, MF, Burton, CR and Watkins, CL (2008) Engaging service users in the development of stroke services: an action research study. *Journal of Clinical Nursing*, 17: 1270–79.

Kai, J, Beavan, J, Faull, C, Dodson, L, Gill, P and Beighton, A (2007) Professional uncertainty and disempowerment. Responding to ethnic diversity in health care: A qualitative study. *PLoS Medicine*, 4(11):1766–74.

Keighley, T and Williams, S (2011) Regulating nursing qualifications across Europe: a case of unintended consequences. *Eurohealth*, 17(4): 11–13.

Kendall-Raynor, P (2012) Scepticism over plans to reward hospitals that use NHS safety tool. *Nursing Standard*, 26(20): 10.

Kennedy, I (2001) *Learning from Bristol: the report of the public inquiry into children's heart surgery at the Bristol Royal Infirmary 1984–1995*. Available at: www.bristol-inquiry.org.uk.

Kenny, G (2002) Interprofessional working: opportunities and challenges. *Nursing Standard*, 17(6): 33–35.

Kilbride, C, Perry, L, Flatley, M, Turner, E and Meyer, J (2011) Developing theory and practice: creation of a Community of Practice through action research produced excellence in stroke care. *Journal of Interprofessional Care*, 25: 91–7.

Klein, R (1980) Models of man and models of policy: reflections on *Exit, Voice, and Loyalty* ten years later. *Milbank Memorial Fund Quarterly/Health and Society*, 58(3): 416–29.

Klein, R (1984) The politics of participation, in Maxwell, RJ and Weaver, N (eds) *Public participation in health: towards a clearer view*. London: King Edward's Hospital Fund for London.

Kohn, LT, Corrigan, JM and Donaldson, MS (eds) (2000) *To err is human: building a safer health system*. Washington DC: National Academic Press.

Learning Disability Advisory Group (2001) Report to the National Assembly for Wales. *Fulfilling the promises*. Available at: www.assemblywales.org/3bd5365d0001c81f0000500700000000.pdf

Leathard, A (2000) *Health care provision: past, present and into the 21st century* (2nd edn). Cheltenham: Nelson Thornes.

Leathard, A (ed.) (2003) *Interprofessional collaboration: from policy to practice in health and social care*. London: Routledge.

Lees, C (2011) Measuring the patient experience. *Nurse Researcher*, 19(1): 25–8.

Leonard, M, Graham, S and Bonacum, D (2004) The human factor: the critical importance of effective teamwork and communication in providing safe care. *Quality and Safety in Health Care*, 13(Suppl 1): i85-i90.

Leppard, D (2002) Official: Shipman murdered 166 of his patients. *The Sunday Times*, 14 July: 1.

Lewis, J (2001) Older people and the health-social care boundary in the UK: half a century of hidden policy conflict. *Social Policy & Administration*, 35(4): 343–59.

Liefooghe, R, Michiels, N, Habib, S, Moran, MB and De Muynck, A (1995) Perception and social consequences of tuberculosis: a focus group study of tuberculosis patients in Sialkot, Pakistan. *Social Science & Medicine*, 41(12): 1685–92.

Lipsky, M (1980) *Street-level bureaucracy: dilemmas of the individual in public services*. New York: Russell Sage.

Lipson, JG and DeSantis, LA (2007) Current approaches to integrating elements of cultural competence in nursing education. *Journal of Transcultural Nursing*, 18(1): 10S–20S.

Litva, A, Coast, J, Donovan, J, Eyles, J, Shepherd, M, Tacchi, J, Abelson, J and Morgan, K (2002) 'The public is too subjective': public involvement at different levels of health-care decision making. *Social Science & Medicine*, 54: 1825–37.

London Health Observatory (2010) *Jubilee line of health inequality*. Available at: www.lho.org.uk/view Resource.aspx?id=15463.

Maben, J and Griffiths, P (2008) *Nurses in society: starting the debate*. National Nursing Research Unit, King's College London, University of London.

Macintyre, S (1997) The Black Report and beyond. What are the issues? *Social Science & Medicine*, 44(6): 723–45.

Marmot, M (1996) The social pattern of health and disease, in Blane, D, Brunner, E and Wilkinson, R (eds) *Health and social organisation: towards a health policy for the twenty-first century*. London: Routledge.

Marmot, M (1999) Introduction, in Marmot, M and Wilkinson, RG (eds) *Social determinants of health*. Oxford: Oxford University Press.

Marmot, MG and Davey Smith, G (1997) Socio-economic differentials in health: the contribution of the Whitehall Studies. *Journal of Health Psychology*, 2(3): 283–96.

Marmot Review (2010) *Fair society, healthy lives. The Marmot Review Executive Summary. Strategic Review of Health Inequalities in England post-2010*. London: The Marmot Review. Available at: www.instituteofhealthequity. org/projects/fair-society-healthy-lives-the-marmot-review.

Marshall, TH (1964) Citizenship and social class, in Marshall, TH *Class, citizenship and social development*. New York: Doubleday & Co.

Mason, T and Whitehead, E (2003) *Thinking nursing*. Maidenhead: Open University Press.

McIver, S (1998) Public involvement in the NHS, in Spurgeon, P (ed.) *The new face of the NHS* (2nd edn). London: Royal Society of Medicine.

Meads, G and Ashcroft, J (2005) Introduction, in Meads, G and Ashcroft, J with Barr, H, Scott, R and Wild, A *The case for interprofessional collaboration in health and social care*. Oxford: Blackwell.

Mechanic, D and Meyer, S (2000) Concepts of trust among patients with serious illness. *Social Science & Medicine*, 51: 657–68.

MENCAP (2007) *Death by indifference: following up the Treat me Right! Report*. London: MENCAP. Available at: www.mencap.org.uk/sites/default/files/documents/2008-03/DBIreport.pdf.

Milewa, T, Valentine, J and Calnan, M (1998) Managerialism and active citizenship in Britain's reformed health service: power and community in an era of decentralisation. *Social Science & Medicine*, 47: 507–17.

Milewa, T, Valentine, J and Calnan, M (1999) Community participation and citizenship in British health care planning: narratives of power and involvement in the changing welfare state. *Sociology of Health and Illness*, 21(4): 445–65.

Miliband, E (2012) Everyone who loves the NHS must fight to defeat this bill. *The Observer*, 5 February: 8.

Milligan, C, Roberts, C and Mort, M (2011) Telecare and older people. Who cares where? *Social Science & Medicine*, 72: 347–54.

Milligan, F and Dennis, S (2004) Improving patient safety and incident reporting. *Nursing Standard*, 19(7): 33–6.

Möllering, G (2001) The nature of trust: From Georg Simmel to a theory of expectation, interpretation and suspension. *Sociology*, 35(2): 403–20.

MORI Social Research Institute (2003) *Exploring trust in public institutions: report for the Audit Commission*. London: MORI Social Research Institute.

Mossialos, E, Permanand, G, Baeten, R and Hervey, T (eds) (2010) *Health systems governance in Europe: the role of European law and policy*. Cambridge: Cambridge University Press.

Muecke, MA (1992) Nursing research with refugees: a review and guide. *Western Journal of Nursing Research*, 14(6): 703–20.

Muir Gray, JA (2004) *Evidence-based healthcare* (2nd edn.). Edinburgh: Churchill Livingstone.

Nazroo, JY (1997) *The health of Britain's ethnic minorities*. London: Policy Studies Institute.

Nazroo, JY (1998) Genetic, cultural or socio-economic vulnerability? Explaining ethnic inequalities in health. *Sociology of Health and Illness*, 20(5): 710–30.

NHS Commissioning Board (2012a) *Arrangements to secure children's and adult safeguarding in the future NHS*. Available at: www.commissioningboard.nhs.uk/files/2012/09/interim-safeguarding.pdf.

NHS Commissioning Board (2012b) Developing our culture of compassionate care: creating a new vision for nurses, midwives and care-givers. Available at: www.commissioningboard.nhs.uk/2012/10/17/comp-care-jc/.

NHS Institute for Innovation and Improvement (2011) *Productive Ward*. Available at: www.institute.nhs.uk/quality_and_value/productivity_series/the_productive_series.html.

NHS London (2012) News Release. NHS London names preferred universities for teaching nurses and physiotherapists the right skills to improve patient care. Tuesday 17 January. London: NHS London. Available at: www.mynhsalerts.london.nhs.uk/2012/01/nhs-london-names-preferred-universities-for-teaching-nurses-and-physiotherapists-skills-to-improve-patient-care/.

NHSE (NHS Executive) (1996) *Patient partnership: building a collaborative strategy*. Leeds: NHSE.

NHSE (1999) *Clinical governance: quality in the new NHS*. Norwich: The Stationery Office.

NHSME (National Health Service Management Executive) (1992) *Local voices: involving the local community in purchasing solutions*. Leeds: NHSME.

NICE (National Institute for Health and Clinical Excellence) (2004) *CSGSP: improving supportive and palliative care*. Available at: http://guidance.nice.org.uk/CSGSP/Guidance/pdf/English.

NICE (2006a) *CG43. Obesity: guidance on the prevention, identification, assessment and management of overweight and obesity in adults and children*. Available at: www.nice.org.uk/guidance/CG43.

NICE (2006b) *CG32. Nutrition support in adults: oral nutrition support, enteral tube feeding and parenteral nutrition*. Available at: www.nice.org.uk/guidance/CG32.

NICE (2007) *CG50. Acutely ill patients in hospital: recognition of and response to acute illness in adults in hospital*. Available at: www.nice.org.uk/guidance/CG50.

NICE (2008) *CG68. Stroke: diagnosis and initial management of acute stroke and transient ischaemic attack (TIA)*. Available at: www.nice.org.uk/guidance/CG68.

NICE (2011) *Tuberculosis: clinical diagnosis and management of tuberculosis, and measures for its prevention and control. NICE clinical guideline 117*. Available at: www.nice.org.uk/guidance/CG117.

NICE (2012) *Identifying and managing tuberculosis among hard-to-reach groups*. NICE public health guidance 37. Available at: www.nice.org.uk/ph37.

NICE/SCIE (2006) *Dementia: supporting people with dementia and their carers in health and social care*. Norwich: The Stationery Office.

NMC (2008) *The code: standards of conduct, performance and ethics for nurses and midwives*. London: NMC.

NMC (2009) *Guidance for the care of older people*. London: NMC.

NMC (2010) *Standards for pre-registration nursing education*. London: NMC.

NMC (2011) *NMC response to the EU Commission's Green Paper on modernising the professional qualifications directive*. London: NMC.

NNRU (National Nursing Research Unit) (2012a) Intentional rounding: What is the evidence? *Policy+. Policy plus evidence, issues and opinions in healthcare. Issue 35*. London: National Nursing Research Unit, King's College London. Available at: www.kcl.ac.uk/nursing/research/nnru/publications/Policy-plus-Review.pdf.

NNRU (2012b) Is it time to set minimum staffing levels in English hospitals? *Policy+ Policy plus evidence, issues and opinions in healthcare*. Issue 34, March 2012. London: National Nursing Research Unit.

North, N (1997) Consumers, service users or citizens? in North, N and Bradshaw, Y (eds) *Perspectives in health care*. Basingstoke: Macmillan.

NPSA (National Patient Safety Agency) (2004) *Seven steps to patient safety: an overview guide for NHS staff*. London: National Patient Safety Agency.

NPSA (2007) *Safer care for the acutely ill patient*. London: National Patient Safety Agency.

Nursing Forum (2012) *About the Nursing and Care Quality Forum*. Available at: www.ncqf.dh.gov.uk/aboutncqf.

Nursing Standard (2011) NHS trusts advised to renegotiate 'wasteful' building repayments. *Nursing Standard*, 26(4): 10.

Oliver, D (1993) Citizenship in the 1990s. *Politics Review*, September: 25–8.

Pahor, M and Rasmussen, BH (2009) How does culture show? A case study of an international and interprofessional course in palliative care. *Journal of Interprofessional Care*, 23(5): 474–85.

Pallister, C and Lavin, J (2010) Working together to manage a programme of weight loss. *Primary Health Care*, 20(10): 28–32.

Papadopoulos, I. (2006) The Papadopoulos, Tilki and Taylor model of developing cultural competence, in Papadopoulos, I. (ed.) *Transcultural health and social care; development of culturally competent practitioners.* London: Elsevier.

Parliamentary and Health Service Ombudsman (2009) *Six lives: the provision of public services to people with learning disabilities.* Available at: www.ombudsman.org.uk/improving-public-service/reports-and-consultations/ reports/health/six-lives-the-provision-of-public-services-to-people-with-learning-disabilities.

Parliamentary and Health Service Ombudsman (2011) *Care and compassion? Reports of the Health Service Ombudsman on ten investigations into NHS care of older people.* London: The Stationery Office.

Patients Association (2011) *We've been listening, have you been learning?* London: The Patients Association.

Perkins, N, Penhale, B, Reid, D, Pinkney, L, Hussein, S and Manthorpe, J (2007) Partnership means protection? Perceptions of the effectiveness of multi-agency working and the regulatory framework within England and Wales. *The Journal of Adult Protection*, 9(3): 9–23.

Phillimore, J (2010) Approaches to health provision in the age of super-diversity: Accessing the NHS in Britain's most diverse city. *Critical Social Policy*, 31(1): 5–29.

Phillips, L (2012) Improving care for people with learning disabilities in hospital. *Nursing Standard*, 26(23): 42–48.

Pollard, K, Sellman, D and Senior, B (2005) The need for interprofessional working, in Barrett, G, Sellman, D and Thomas, J *Interprofessional working in health and social care.* London: Routledge.

Pollock, AM and Price, D (2011) How the secretary of state for health proposes to abolish the NHS in England. *British Medical Journal*, 342: d1695.

Pollock, AM, Price, D, Roderick, P, Treuherz, T, McCoy, D, McKee, M and Reynolds, L (2012) How the Health and Social Care Bill 2011 would end entitlement to comprehensive health care in England. *The Lancet*, 379(9814): 387–9.

Powell, J, Gunn, L, Lowe, P, Sheehan, B, Griffiths, F and Clarke, A (2010) New networked technologies and carers of people with dementia: an interview study. *Ageing & Society*, 30(6): 1073–88.

Prior, D, Stewart, J and Walsh, K (1995) *Citizenship: rights, community and participation.* London: Pitman.

Rawls, J (1972) *A theory of justice.* Oxford: Clarendon Press.

RCN (Royal College of Nursing) (2010) *Response to the NHS White Paper: Equity and excellence: Liberating the NHS (England).* London: RCN.

RCN (2011a) *The RCN and the Health and Social Care Bill.* London: RCN.

RCN (2011b) *Time to care.* London: RCN.

RCN (2012a) Results of RCN member vote on pensions, 28 February. Available at: www.rcn.org.uk/ newsevents/news/article/uk/results_of_rcn_member_vote_on_pensions (accessed 29 February 2012).

RCN (2012b) *Position statement on the education and training of health care assistants (HCAs).* London: RCN.

RCN (2012c) *Safe staffing for older people's wards. RCN summary guidance and recommendations.* London: RCN.

Reason, J (1990) *Human error.* Cambridge: Cambridge University Press.

Rees, AM (1995) The promise of social citizenship. *Policy and Politics*, 23 (4): 313–25.

Richardson, A, Sitzia, J and Cotterell, P (2005) 'Working the system': achieving change through partnership working: an evaluation of cancer partnership groups. *Health Expectations*, 8: 210–20.

Roach, MS (2002) *Caring, the human mode of being: a blueprint for the health professions* (second revised edn). Ottawa: CH Press.

Rowe, R and Calnan, M (2006) Trust relations in health care: developing a theoretical framework for the 'new' NHS. *Journal of Health Organization & Management*, 20(5): 376–96.

RCP (Royal College of Physicians) (2012a) *National Early Warning Score (NEWS).* London: RCP. Available at: www.rcplondon.ac.uk/resources/national-early-warning-score-news.

RCP (2012b) *Hospitals on the edge? The time for action.* London: RCP.

RCP and RCN (Royal College of Physicians and Royal College of Nursing) (2012) *Ward rounds in medicine: principles for best practice.* London: RCP.

Royal College of Psychiatrists (2010) *No health without public mental health: the case for action. Position statement PS4/2010.* London: Royal College of Psychiatrists.

Rummery, K (2009) Health partnerships, healthy citizens? An international review of partnerships in health and social care and patient/user outcomes. *Social Science & Medicine*, 69(12): 1797–804.

Sample, I (2012) Omega-3 may help struggling children to read, says study. *The Guardian*, 6 September.

Sampson, EL, Candy, B and Jones, J (2009) There is insufficient evidence to suggest that enteral tube feeding is beneficial in patients with advanced dementia. *Cochrane Summaries. Cochrane Database*. Available at: http://summaries.cochrane.org/CD007209 (accessed 23 October 2012).

Scott, I (1999) Clinical governance: An opportunity for nurses to influence the future of healthcare development. *Nursing Times Research*, 4(3): 170–6.

Scott, R, Ashcroft, J and Wild, A (2005) Crisis prevention, in Meads, G and Ashcroft, J with Barr, H, Scott, R and Wild, A *The case for interprofessional collaboration in health and social care*. Oxford: Blackwell.

Scottish Executive (2000) *The same as you? A review of services for people with learning disabilities*. Available at: www.scotland.gov.uk/Resource/Doc/1095/0001661.pdf.

Secretary of State for Health (2007) *Trust, assurance and safety: the regulation of health professionals in the 21st century*. Cm 7013. London: The Stationery Office.

Sevenhuijsen, S (2000) Caring in the third way: the relation between obligation, responsibility and care in Third Way discourse. *Critical Social Policy*, 20 (5): 5–37.

Shaw, M, Davey Smith, G and Dorling, D (2005) Health inequalities and New Labour: how the promises compare with real progress. *British Medical Journal*, 330: 1016–21.

Slowther, A, Hundt, GL, Taylor, R and Purkis, J (2009) *Non UK qualified doctors and good medical practice: the experience of working within a different professional framework. Report for the General Medical Council*. Coventry: University of Warwick.

Smaje, C (1995) *Health, 'race' and ethnicity: making sense of the evidence*. London: King's Fund.

Smith, E and Ross, FM (2007) Service user involvement and integrated care pathways. *International Journal of Health Care Quality Assurance*, 20(3): 195–214.

Smith, PA, Allan, H, Henry, LW, Larsen, JA and Mackintosh, MM (2006) *Valuing and recognising the talents of a diverse healthcare workforce*. London: Royal College of Nursing.

Smithers, R (2012) Health warning on salt levels in bacon. *The Guardian*, Thursday 13 September.

Steenbergen, B van (ed.) (1994) *The condition of citizenship*. London: Sage.

Stiglitz, JE, Sen, A and Fitoussi, J (2009) *Report by the Commission on the Measurement of Economic Performance and Social Progress*. Available at www.stiglitz-sen-fitoussi.fr.

Sturgeon, D (2008) Measuring compassion in nursing. *Nursing Standard*, 22(46): 42–3.

Summerfield, D (1999) Sociocultural dimensions of war, conflict and displacement, in Ager, A (ed.) *Refugees: perspectives on the experience of forced migration*. London: Cassell.

Swinkels, A and Mitchell, T (2008) Delayed transfer from hospital to community settings: the older person's perspective. *Health and Social Care in the Community*, 17(1): 45–53.

Taylor, G (2007) An investigation into the health-related quality of life of refugees and asylum seekers in Britain and France (unpublished PhD thesis). London: Middlesex University.

Taylor, G, Wangaruro, J and Papadopoulos, I (2012) 'It is my turn to give': migrants' maintenance of transnational identity. *Journal of Ethnic & Migration Studies*, 38(7): 1085–100.

Templeton, S (2011) Nurses want relatives to care for sick. *The Sunday Times*, 25 September: 1.

Templeton, S (2012a) Parents found girl, 12, in rigor mortis in NHS bed. *The Sunday Times*, 5 August: 12.

Templeton, S (2012b) A sip of water might have kept Mum alive. *The Sunday Times*, 22 July: 11.

Thaler, RH and Sunstein, CR (2009) *Nudge: improving decisions about health, wealth and happiness*. London: Penguin Books.

Thompson, I E, Melia, KM, Boyd, KM and Horsburgh, D (2006) *Nursing ethics* (5th edn). Edinburgh: Churchill Livingstone.

Timmins, N (1994) Christopher Clunis Report: schizophrenic made 'series of violent attacks'. *The Independent*, 25 February.

Titmuss, RM (1970) *The Gift Relationship: from human blood to social policy*. London: George Allen & Unwin.

Titmuss, RM (1974) Postscript, in Abel-Smith, B and Titmuss, J (eds) *Social policy: an introduction*. London: George Allen & Unwin.

Townsend, P, Davidson, N and Whitehead, M (1992) *Inequalities in health* (2nd edn). Harmondsworth: Penguin.

Triggle, N (2012) Nursing standards: PM aims to tackle 'care problem'. *BBC News*. Health, 6 January. Available at: www.bbc.co.uk/news/health-16425043 (accessed 6 January 2012).

Ungerson, C (1987) *Policy is personal*. London: Tavistock.

Unwin, N, Carr, S, Leeson, J and Pless-Mulloli, T (1997) *An introductory study guide to public health and epidemiology*. Buckingham: Open University Press.

Wenger, D (1998) *Communities of practice: learning, meaning and identity*. Cambridge: Cambridge University Press.

West, E and Scott, C (2000) Nursing in the public sphere: breaching the boundary between research and policy. *Journal of Advanced Nursing*, 32: 817–24.

WHO (2009a) *Global priorities for patient safety research: better knowledge for safer care*. Geneva: WHO.

WHO (2009b) *WHO guidelines on hand hygiene in health care*. Geneva: WHO.

WHO (2010) *Strategic directions for strengthening nursing and midwifery service 2011–2015*. Geneva: WHO.

WHO (2011) *Patient safety curriculum guide: multi-professional education*. Geneva: WHO.

WHO (2012) *Patient safety*. Available at: www.who.int/patientsafety/about/en/index.html.

WHO Regional Office for Europe (2012) *Health 2020: a European policy framework supporting action across government and society for health and well-being*. Copenhagen: WHO Regional Office for Europe.

Wilkinson, RG (1992) Income distribution and life expectancy. *British Medical Journal*, 304: 165–8.

Wilkinson, RG (1996) *Unhealthy societies: the afflictions of inequality*. London: Routledge.

Wilson, PM (2001) A policy analysis of the expert patient in the United Kingdom: self-care as an expression of pastoral power? *Health and Social Care in the Community*, 9(3): 134–42.

Woodward, S (2006) Learning and sharing safety lessons to improve patient care. *Nursing Standard*, 20(18): 49–53.

Yang, LH, Kleinman, A, Link, BG, Phelan, JC, Lee, S and Good, B (2007) Culture and stigma: adding moral experience to stigma theory. *Social Science & Medicine*, 64: 1524–35.

Index